HYPNOTIC WOMEN

Present a Collection of Therapeutic Stories, Scripts, Poems and Inductions

Edited by Kelley T. Woods

Disclaimer

The contents of this book are for information purposes only and the contributors and publisher do not accept any responsibilities for any liabilities resulting from the use of this information. Content contained herein is presented as original material by the individual contributors and the publisher takes no responsibility for verity of such claim.

The hypnotic approaches described in this book are not a substitute for medical treatment; practitioners are not diagnosing or treating any medical or psychiatric disorders and it is recommended that a medical referral is procured before working with clients who present with such issues.

TABLE OF CONTENTS

Chapter		Page

Foreword

by Dr. Fred H. Janke

I am very pleased and honored to be asked to provide a forward for what I consider a unique and useful resource for all hypnotherapists. My interest in hypnotherapy began a number of years ago when I became frustrated with not having more to offer patients who were suffering with chronic pain. For many such patients there is often a never-ending spiral of pain, disability, medication, dependence and illness roles. I began to explore complementary therapies and soon began to realize that hypnotherapy had so much to offer. A well-trained and skilled hypnotherapist could not only help directly with the pain, but also with the emotional consequences related to chronic illness. With further research into hypnotherapy I began to realize the vast scope of clinical domains for which it could be applied. I also began to understand that the successful application of hypnosis to clinical problems very much depends on the training and skill of the "operator."

My search for an experienced professional led me to Sherry Hood and her school, The Pacific Institute of Advanced Hypnotherapy. Our first project together was a small research study on smoking cessation. We were able to have a "Poster" accepted at the Alberta Scientific Assembly of the Alberta College of Family Physicians presenting our results. This small study displayed the potential of hypnotherapy showing a long-term success rate at least as good as the medications being used for smoking cessation. Hypnotherapy had other positive outcomes, such as a decrease in anxiety, whereas medications are encumbered with a variety of side effects. We continue to seek funding to conduct a larger broader study.

Since that research study, Sherry and I have embarked on many projects together including joint authorship on a number of articles and joint workshop presentations at medical conferences. These projects have required us to complete fairly rigorous literature reviews and in turn I have become familiar with some of the scientific literature and research pertaining to hypnotherapy. It is a fascinating field to study.

I always feel a sense of joy to see the amazement on medical student's faces, when I show a video clip of surgery being done completely under hypnosis and no anesthetic. As the students reflect, they gain insight into the vast amount of cost savings such an approach could have in our health care system.

The understanding around hypnotherapy and its many uses in complementary medicine has grown considerably over the last number of decades. Imaging studies including MRI and PET scanning have helped gain a better understanding as to where in the brain, hypnosis has its effects. Other research studies, including randomized controlled trials have helped build the evidence regarding the effectiveness of hypnotherapy in many clinical areas. Much more remains to be done. Good research in hypnotherapy is difficult. Design of studies is challenged by the fact that it is difficult to find a placebo control. It is also difficult to adequately "blind" volunteers to being in a hypnotherapy group versus being in a control group. We know that simply being in a study often has its own effects on the study population. Thus research studies in hypnotherapy are often small, not well designed and they vary widely in their results. Although challenging, good studies are possible and we need so many more.

"Hypnotic Women" was the brainchild of Kelley T. Woods who was seeking to find a supportive network among fellow women hypnotherapists. The network has grown exponentially and presently hosts about 300 members. A supportive network like this allows one to not only share ideas and experiences, but allows creativity and innovation by bouncing brainstorming ideas off one another.

It was Sherry Hood's idea to collect hypnotherapy scripts from members and collate them into a collection that has resulted in this book. The concept was to share and learn from each other and then to share with others.

This book is unique in many ways. The scripts have come only from members and thereby represent the work of female hypnotherapists. I believe women often have a special way of looking at concerns and issues, call it a special form of emotional intelligence that we men often lack. Women also often have a unique way of connecting with hurting individuals. The scripts found in this book are the insights of professional women as they embark on helping their clients. The authors hope that their contributions will help others by providing an insight into the wide variety of ways or approaches a script can be designed and written.

The scripts were submitted without being directed to a specific topic or clinical area. Therefore each contributor has written from her own interests and passions. Quite a wide variety of topics are covered. Where topics overlap, the scripts provide different perspectives and different approaches to the same type of problem.

Another unique aspect of the book is that contributors vary considerably in their experience and field of work. Some of the scripts have been submitted by students, some by recent graduates yet others by highly experienced and skilled professionals. I find particular joy in this. Everyone has something unique to offer and in my own work I find I often learn as much (perhaps more) from my students as they learn from me.

I am very excited to see this collection come together in one compilation. I feel very confident that that many hypnotherapists will find it not only useful but also very interesting. Please enjoy.

Dr. Janke completed his degree in medicine at the University of Calgary in 1982 and has been practicing in Sylvan Lake, Alberta, Canada as a family physician since 1984.

He became involved with the University of Alberta as site director in Red Deer for a new rural stream family medicine residency program in the year 2000. Since then he has become increasingly involved with teaching family medicine at the postgraduate level. In 2008, he took on the role of "Rural Program Director," in the Department of Family Medicine at the University of Alberta. In that role he became full time faculty, although his clinical work remains in Sylvan Lake. He is the first "geographic full time equivalent" member in the Faculty of Medicine to have his home base and clinical practice outside of Edmonton. He became Director of Rural and Regional Health in the Division of Community Engagement in 2011.

Dr. Janke has been recognized through a number of awards including "Outstanding Clinician of the Year" for the David Thompson Health Region in the year 2000, Family Physician Fellowship Award from the College of Family Physicians of Canada in 2002 and an award for excellence in clinical teaching in the year 2002/3. He also received Citizen of the Year Award in Sylvan Lake in the year 2000. In 2009 he received a Fellowship from the Society of Rural Physicians of Canada in recognition of his contributions to rural medicine.

Introduction

"There are women who make things better...simply by showing up. There are women who make things happen. There are women who make their way. There are women who make a difference. And women who make us smile. There are women of wit and wisdom who - through strength and courage - make it through. There are women who change the world every day...Women like you."
~ Ashley Rice

The sentiments in the quote above are what inspired this collaboration of works written by 57 females working primarily in hypnosis. Whether you are a male or a female hypnosis practitioner, we thank you for purchasing and supporting our cause. (All profits are designated toward educational scholarships for Hypnotic Women.)

The benefits of social media are evident in how the contributors of this tome were not only connected, but were inspired to participate in this project. In today's world, it's no longer necessary to operate in isolation as a private hypnosis practitioner; we are now easily able to access numerous resources, lifting our perspectives, abilities and our spirits.

This is a precious field and the community that it creates is unique and beautiful. Hypnotists and hypnotherapists are drawn to this work because they want to make a difference; they want to facilitate healing and empowerment in others and they have a genuine desire to help humanity.

As the field of Hypnotherapy continues to grow, practitioners are dedicated to a high standard of practice in facilitating empowerment and healing with their clients. This includes quality education with a broad scope of learning and ongoing, up-to-date continuing education and mentoring. Sharing ideas and resources like the ones contained in this book helps inspire us all to combine creativity and science while promoting transformative change.

Hypnotic Women is a result of like-minded individuals who are passionately working together with the same vision. In order to allow a free flow of creative expression, topics were not assigned to authors and women submitted scripts, poems and information that they hold close to their hearts. The dynamic, intuitive power of the female spirit comes through in the contents of this book. It has been a joy to put it together and we expect that you will find that reading and applying the wonderful collection to your work and life to be a rewarding experience.

We wish you much happiness and success in all that you do!

Kelley T. Woods and *Sherry M. Hood*

Chapter 1   Rapid Inductions

Have Fun, Increase Confidence, and Build Rapport with Rapid Inductions

by Cindy Levy

I love how hypnosis feels, especially when it occurs rapidly. Dropping into trance feels like sliding down into a soft, velvety nest at the center of my being. I hope to feel that when someone else leads me into hypnosis, and I hope to create an experience for my clients that feels similar, or equally as good, according to their representational systems (visual, auditory, and/or kinesthetic). As you can tell, mine is kinesthetic in this context.

Everyone goes into trance. It is hard-wired into our brains, as a neuro-biological necessity. Our brainwaves cycle throughout the day in roughly 90 – 120 minute intervals. The waking state is characterized by beta waves, and lighter trance/daydreaming states by alpha waves, and deeper trance/full immersive states by theta waves. This periodic cycling is a homeostatic mechanism which helps maintain brain health.

As hypnotists, we are detectives exploring how each person manifests their ability to go into trance, as well as their understanding of their own process. We want to know how our clients describe to themselves what "altered states" they have experienced. We then use the client's words to first educate them about what hypnosis is by relating it to the phenomena they just described, then leading them intentionally to that state, in a way that meets their understandings and expectations. When that happens, the client can more readily believe they were "hypnotized".

A way to strengthen that belief is to use what we call convincers. These are physical phenomena which demonstrate automatic subconscious responses, independent of conscious volition. Combining convincers with phenomena the clients already knows has the effect of pacing their current experience, and leading them to greater innate abilities they don't yet know. This generates curiosity, opens their mind more, deepens the trance, strengthens rapport, and further establishes your expertise.

A rapid induction almost always has a convincer, and is a convincer in itself. Rapids work well for people new to hypnosis, as well as for experienced subjects. In fact, people experienced with hypnosis usually want to enter back in quickly, and are bored with long, drawn-out inductions such as progressive muscle relaxation. Boredom isn't fun, but quick and instant hypnosis is. And, in our busy lives, we can more easily take 5 – 10 min. total for a timeout to drop down, feel good, refresh, then get back into the day.

For people new to hypnosis, a rapid induction with convincers has the "Wow!" factor. True hypnotic phenomena is actually happening! Their eyes are stuck shut! Their arm is actually raising or lowering! Their hands are clasped shut! Their arm is rigid! Then, their arm collapses, and gets so relaxed they don't want to move it! That's crazy! Yet, it's happening. And, if they really wanted to, they could [try to] stop it, but they don't want to! What's up with that!?

This creates confusion and overwhelm. The reason this

successfully results in a positive trance state is due to the trust and rapport you build, and your skillful holding of the person which allows them to enter unknown territory. Their subjective experience is an edge of anxiety co-existing with the "Cool!" factor, as they discover more of their capabilities. It is a privilege to facilitate this, and exciting to witness.

The more you do this, the more confident you become. It doesn't take long before you discover a secret: most people are hungry for this. They want a skillful, trustworthy operator to introduce them to the wonders that lie within their own minds. They want to awaken their awareness, tap their abilities, stretch themselves, be creative, and live up to the potential they sense inside themselves. When someone like you comes along, their insides say, "Yes!" What you need most now is to believe you will deliver on that promise. Of course, you won't do the work for them. All you'll do is lead the horse to water. They'll feel the thirst in themselves.

Have you experienced a rapid induction for yourself? I highly recommend it. Ask another hypnotist to do one with you – chances are, they'll be happy to. Ask to learn it, and practice it with them. Then, seek out other opportunities. It's not hard. Many people are curious and eager.

One rapid induction I like is the rigid arm, or arm catalepsy, where the arm is stiff and unbendable. Suggest that the first time you test it, it's rigid. Then, on the second time, the arm collapses and the person collapses their entire body, loose and limp, and falls deeply into trance. It's a quick, intense experience – and, it releases endorphins. That's a nice side benefit from just an induction. By the way, this is also why hypnosis is good for treating addictions – we can be taught to tap into our inner pharmacy to create our own well-being.

This isn't just exchanging one addiction for another – it's a process of self-empowerment, while healing from chemical dependency.

So, do rapids. Have fun. Show your stuff. Give 'em a "Wow!" experience which feels great, and gives them a taste of what they can do. What greater contribution can we make than by sparking one's excitement for vibrant well-being and the endless possibilities they can create? This makes life an adventure and a playground to be explored. Knowing this, we can make our lives richer, happier, healthier, and more satisfying and meaningful.

The Client Enters Your Room

by Joanna Cameron

"Anecdotes, one-liners and analogies do not merely energize therapy and make ideas memorable; they are also used to guide associations. Problems are often caused by preconscious associations. If problems are generated at the level of associations, it often is at that level that they can best be changed. Anecdotes can be used to help reassociate the patient's internal life. Merely talking about a situation is not necessarily therapeutic."

~ Milton Erickson

CHANGE is the operative word. That's what our clients want. That is what we want for them. So we must "lay the table, set the stage, provide the atmosphere" with **CHANGE** in mind. I have a lazy boy chair and a couch in my office, so as I open the door, I say:

*"Welcome to the hypnochange room! You can sit in either chair for a **change**. Do you want to **change now or change later?**" (the client may pull an odd face...so LAUGH!!)*

Obviously, I obtain needed information from the client. However, as I do this, I use classic rapport techniques: mirroring the client's body language, identifying the client's representational system (are they visual, kinesthetic, auditory etc?) and feeding their words back to them. When you are in rapport, you will know it...*just feel it*. And it is a bonus when the client says something like, "You know, I feel like I have known you for a long time...."

Now it is your turn to lead:

You want the client to follow your lead. My friend, Justin Tranz, calls this *"going through the hoops."* On the stage, it involves dancing, clapping, even chanting or singing (and I have done this in my office). I think suggestibility tests in the office are fun and please do them with the client standing up.

Here's the most important thing: **Never give up your power**. *Never* mention, *"I cannot make you do anything that you don't want to do."* Ooh, I hate even typing that sentence!

"Hypnosis is simply accepting a suggestion – come on now – that's what you want. That's why you are here. Let's face it – we learn by accepting suggestions. You have come here because your own thoughts are not working. So it's time for some new thoughts!! Yeah!!! It is time to open up the magic of your mind. (Get some excitement!). Now, only about 5% of the population has been hypnotized by a therapist so most of my clients are experiencing it for the first time – so no worries. I cannot (shake your head) *make you rob a bank and you are not going to give me your ATM pin* (laugh and the client will laugh also.) *So are you ready to be hypnotized..."* Get a yes. If the client ever asks you if they will reveal secrets, just shake your head, laugh and **don't look** at them (too threatening).

To watch the Trance Lady in action, you can see my video: www.youtube.com/watch?v=Q_7QqfmwEg8

Conscious/Unconscious Dissociation
(The Confusion Technique)

Analytical-computer-type-digital-processing-clients may be listening to their own self-talk rather than focusing on what the hypnotherapist is saying. I find that confusion works really well in these cases.

Overload = Ambiguity = Trance

So you separate the attention and intention of the conscious versus the unconscious mind. Most people cannot operate in this split awareness without overload.

You can start with either Conversational Induction (1) or (2) and if you need to, go into this Confusion Technique. Remember, it does not matter if it makes sense or not as the whole idea is just overload.

"Your conscious mind can just go ahead and sit there and pay attention to that spot on the wall, or listen to the sound of my voice, because I'm not interested in talking to your conscious mind. I'm interested in talking to **your unconscious** mind. And **your unconscious** mind can do many things that your conscious mind is not aware of...like your conscious mind doesn't usually know when your eyes are going to blink because **your unconscious** mind can blink those eyes. And your conscious mind can only wander as **your unconscious** mind wonders. And **your unconscious** mind can remember those things that your conscious mind may forget, and **your conscious** mind can remember to forget those things that **your unconscious** mind remembers. And I wonder if your conscious mind can remember to remember to forget those things which **your unconscious mind** remembers..."

Post Hypnotic Suggestions

The Amnesia Sandwich

I use indirect techniques/conversational techniques to induce trance but once trance has been established there is nothing quite like a direct suggestion given within an amnesia sandwich. This way the conscious mind does not analyze the suggestion. A post-hypnotic suggestion is any command given during a hypnotic session that modifies a behavior after the hypnotic session is over.

"Every time you wake up in the morning you know that you are a non-smoker."

"Every time you have a fork in your hand, you remember to eat slowly and your metabolism will increase to whatever level is most effective for you to digest your food easily and effortlessly..."

Induce trance. Tell a story or use a metaphor(s). Then deepen the trance. I like fractionation, a staircase...elevator.

At this point, amnesia should be introduced. Amnesia is the deepest part of the hypnotic session. It is easily accomplished by radically changing the subject and associating the client to previous times when they successfully accomplished amnesia.

"When you have a meal, you can be really satisfied at the end of the meal, but you don't have to review every piece or every nutrient you've consumed. Forgetting is a natural and normal state. Come to think of it, I don't remember what I had for lunch last Thursday... However, it doesn't mean that it is gone. In fact, it means that it went way

*down into **your unconscious**, so deep that you have consciously forgotten the information. And your conscious mind can remember to forget those things that **your unconscious** mind remembers..."*

(Now give the suggestion: *You are a non smoker.*). Then talk about forgetting again, *"You know I really don't remember the last time that I smoked was in a hot tub. But maybe you know how hard it is to smoke in a hot tub or on a ski hill for that matter – with the wind blowing, and those mittens."*

When working with amnesia give more suggestions of relaxation; this inherently creates trance within a trance...

At the end of the therapy, give the client suggestions of self-appreciation. This will assist alignment between the conscious and unconscious minds. It also increases the client's self-esteem by providing the opportunity for conscious appreciation of the client's abilities, intent, essence, spirit etc.

"The more I do hypnotherapy, the more I believe that we must spend most of our time with the client visualizing, feeling, hearing and energizing the future. Many of our clients are stuck in the past. We must shift that awareness to the future. We must teach our clients to DREAM. The thoughts we have today will be our tomorrow. So, let's think about something good!" ~ Joanna Cameron

Gentle Rapid Induction Outline

by Lorraine Gleeson

This is an outline and definitely not a script!

This is a technique that I use when I am giving a talk and to demonstrate a technique. It looks quite impressive to the people watching and it is not a shock to the person who has volunteered.

You get the person to take a seat and ask them to take a deep breath and close their eyes. You then take their arm nearest to you (I stand at their side) and lift it right up in the air; you say something along the lines of, *"This is your conscious analytical mind, wide awake and alert."*

I then lean across them and put my four fingers under their wrist on their other hand (which is usually on their lap or on the arm of the chair) you need to push their arm in an upward direction (this does take practice as you want it to look natural). It needs to look as though their other arm starts to go upwards. *"This arm represents your subconscious mind and as this arm comes up, you find you are relaxing more and more..."*

Now they are sitting with their eyes closed and one arm in the air and their other arm is starting to rise. You then tap the top of the other hand (which represents being wide awake) and you start the suggestions.

For example: *"And as your arm comes down you find that you are relaxing and your other arm is getting lighter and lighter, that's right, as you allow yourself to relax, notice that your breathing is slowing down.. that's right, you find yourself just drifting..."*

You continue with the usual hypnotic suggestions, until the light arm has risen right up into the air and the other arm has come down to rest.

At this point I then suggest that as I bring the light arm down (usually I will say that I will count down to five or something) and when this arm reaches your lap you may double that relaxation, and when it touches their lap I may say something like *"That's right, double that relaxation"*.

Instant and Rapid Inductions

by Mariana Matthews

This is not training for instant and rapid inductions but, instead, it is an overview, with tips and safety reminders. Even though this book is meant for those already trained and/or practicing hypnosis, I would suggest that you take in-person Instant and Rapid Induction courses for proper techniques, safety, practice. I have personally trained with three fantastic teachers and am happy to share their contact information with anyone that is interested.

In my opinion, all hypnotists should have this valuable asset in their tool belt. I am a certified hypnotherapist and have specialty certifications in many subjects, but my true passion comes from demonstrating the powers of the mind via Stage Comedy Hypnosis Shows. Instant and Rapid Inductions can be used for lecture demonstrations, therapy sessions, street hypnosis, emergency situations and also for stage. I use them in almost every performance, either as an initial induction or deepener. Instant Inductions are also a great way to select volunteers pre-show.

Safety

Instant and Rapid Inductions provide a WOW factor for both the volunteer and those watching. It sometimes looks violent, but is not, when done properly. Even if done correctly make sure to ALWAYS ask the subject if they have any previous injuries *before* you do the induction. My friend and instant induction mentor, Sean Michael Andrews, teaches the following mnemonic as a safety check:

24

NEWS. It stands for:

- Neck
- Elbow
- Wrist
- Shoulder

Simply ask the subject if they have any injuries to any of the body parts listed above.

When doing a standing induction, make sure your subject has been told that their legs will remain strong, as if they have steel bars in their legs, and that they can stand and sleep, unless your intent is to have them drop to the ground. If so, I advise you have someone nearby to assist or have a chair behind the subject that they can sit on. I recently had a young man (whose English was limited) collapse to the ground, even though I had given the above suggestion. Luckily, he was not a large person and I was able to hold him up until one of his friends assisted me in helping him gently to the ground. This was a crowd pleaser, but not my intent.

Additionally, when performing a standing induction, make sure you and your subject are standing solid, foot position and distance correct...another reason I suggest in-person training and practice.

Overview

There are various ways to induce rapid and instant inductions, but the underlying premise is the same: Our bodies react to external stimuli automatically to keep us safe. A shock, startle, surprise, mental or physical disorientation makes you hyper-alert and extremely suggestible for a brief period of time. If you receive a simple, understandable command during this period of heightened suggestibility, you will execute that command. This is sometimes referred to as the "fright or flight response". In this instance the command is "SLEEP!"

Many of the same elements that are used for any type of induction are important. These are: rapport, consent, induction, deepening and emerging. I find that if my subject understands what will happen, that the induction is almost always successful.

Another important element with an instant or rapid induction is that once the initial bypass of the critical factor is performed, ("*Sleep!*"), subsequent suggestions/deepeners must be given quickly. The language or patter should be simple. I typically start with " *The deeper you go the better you feel. The better you feel the deeper you go*". I also reassure the subject by stating "*that's right*" or "*you are doing great*". This is done as a deepener for a few seconds, after which you can slow down the patter. I also like to lightly rock the individual while tapping the base of the skull while deepening.

Again, like other hypnosis work, convincers are next. Anything like eyes locked, stiff-arm, hand stuck will work. Then proceed to suggestions, which in my case are usually something fun and feel good!

Make sure to emerge your subject, even though we know that they would just pop out of trance within minutes if left on their own. Simply say, "*In a moment, I'm going to ask you to open your eyes feeling alert, refreshed and wonderful. Go ahead and open your eyes.*" Or use your favorite emerging language. This will prevent both volunteers and on-lookers from believing that you left your subjects in trance.

Types of Instant/Rapid Inductions

There are many ways to perform instant and rapid inductions. The style I use depends on the situation, the subject and the location. Also listed is how I use the induction, but again these are just my preferences.

Dave Elman Three Handshake Induction (Modified)

This is one of my favorite Instant Inductions. It is simple and easy for the subject to understand. I use this one for Demonstrations/Lectures usually with the subject standing. I have the advantage of having my husband with me in case my subject is a "flopper". This is an adaptation of a classic Dave Elman induction. The original is simply another version of his famous catalyst induction. This is the way Sean Michael Andrews turns it into a shock induction. *As taught by Sean Michael Andrews*:

Say to your subject, "*I'm going to shake your hand three times. The first time I shake your hand, your eyelids will get heavy and drowsy and you'll want to close them, but don't. The second time I shake your hand, your eyelids will become even more heavy, droopy and drowsy and you'll really want to close them, but don't yet. The third time I shake your hand, your eyelids will close down and lock and you won't be able to open them.* "

Shake the subject's hand. Say, "*Your eyelids become tired, but don't close them yet.*" Shake the subject's hand a second time. "*And now your eyelids are becoming even heavier and you want to close them, but don't.*" Then you do a quick arm

27

pull similar to the one you do in the classic arm pull induction and shout, "*Sleep!*" Deepen immediately.

The following are names of additional Instant and Rapid Inductions which are popular, but the list is by no means all-inclusive.

Hand-drop

I use this for both demonstrations and shows. Always have the subject seated. This induction is one of the most popular, particularly of women. If your subject is larger/ taller/ heavier than you, then this should be your induction of choice. The subject may know that you are going to pull out your hand but will not know *when* which, combined with the shout "*Sleep!*", is the shock which will drop the subject into trance.

Arm-pull I use this one in my shows, subject seated, mainly as a deepener. "*And when I tug on your arm you will go twice as deep as you are now*".

Arm Lock Shock (Steel Arm) I sometimes use this one in my shows as a suggestibility test turned into an Instant Induction.

Handshake Interrupt (I call this one the Creepy Man Handshake) I do not use this because it feels creepy to me...but many like this one.

Pull Neck NOT recommended. Shock induction with hand behind the subject's neck, quick pull of the head towards you.

I would urge you to learn and practice at least one or two instant inductions. I guarantee that you will find it useful.

Chapter 2   Relaxation, Mindfulness, and Meditation

A Full Body Guided Meditation

by Janice Lesley

This is a good meditation for those who enjoy baths over showers. Speak very slowly and allow frequent pauses.

This guided meditation will take you on an imaginary journey and enable you to experience your body in a positive, empowering...and ultimately healing manner.

You do not have to *do anything*...but simply let yourself sink deeply into your chair and relax, and give yourself permission to let go of all your worries and tensions of the day as you do nothing except just simply listen to my voice. And, you don't even need to *try* and do that, because you may instead just drift off and let your mind wander, and if you do, *that's okay,* because a part of your mind will still hear me, and you will still benefit from this lovely, healing guided meditation. So just relax, and let yourself go on this wonderful journey.

Sit back (or lie back) comfortably and close your eyes. Take a few deep breaths and with every breath out, allow yourself to become more relaxed and more at ease...sinking deeper and deeper into a state of calmness and peace...A deep breath in, and a deep breath out, letting tension go and falling *deeper* and *deeper* into a peaceful state, that's right, that's good.

Now, in your imagination or your mind's eye, see yourself in the most beautiful and most comfortable, luxurious master bathroom you have ever seen. Somehow, you know this room has been built specifically to suit you, as the colors are perfect and the spaciousness of the room fits your every need. The huge Jacuzzi tub is situated under a large bay window overlooking a secluded view of greenery with a large expanse of sky. You just know that you would feel so safe here and so private and so relaxed.

You now begin to feel yourself looking forward to a long soak in this huge deep tub as you hear the sound of the water filling up the tub and you note the lovely flower petals floating on the water. There is also a delicate scent of your favorite bubble bath in the room, which you savor as you are slowly preparing to place your clothing on the rich, dark rosewood butler which sits nearby.

You notice that your toes curl up several times as they come into contact with the luxurious carpet beneath your feet. And the temperature of the room feels just right, too, as it is not too cold nor too warm and it feels just perfect for you. You glance around the room and it is either filled with the crisp yellow blue light of day or the deep soothing darkness of starlight, along with candle lights glowing around your tub.

Whatever your choice is, whatever you wish to imagine, it is yours...simply by thinking it so. This is *your special time* and you feel yourself looking forward to becoming even more relaxed as you slowly step into the warm, bubbling water.

Your body becomes fully emerged in the water as you lay back and you find that you can place your head completely and comfortable on a soft pillow. You like this sensation and you close your eyes and let out a big sigh as the warmth of the water begins to sink in. Then, after a while, you open your eyes and they lazily follow the shimmering colors of the bubbles and flower petals as they slowly float by. They are moved by the jets of water that stream from underneath the water and then you notice how these jets are massaging so many different areas of your body, all at the same time. You smile to yourself.

You feel so at ease. The gentle pulses of the radiating water eases your body and you feel yourself releasing any stress you had from the day, and you relax deeper into yourself, almost a sleep-like state. You rest....you relax....You take several deep releasing breaths. Your body feels lulled into a deeper relaxation. The warmth, the aromas, the sensations, all work to envelope you in complete comfort, at just the right temperature. The view is so beautiful and you simply let go...and you rest. You deserve this special time.

Now allow your awareness to notice your toes sticking out of the soapy water. You wiggle them and you begin to think about how important they really are. You feel a growing appreciation for your toes and for what they do for you. You know it is because of your toes that you can balance, as you stand, and that when you move, they give you momentum as they carry you forward in life. And before you are consciously aware of any desire to move at all, you notice that you have brought your left foot forward while your hand is reaching out to that foot and you find yourself touching your toes. You look directly at your toes and say quietly to them, "Thank you, Toes!" and then you notice yourself doing the same thing to your other foot. And you smile gently to yourself.

You feel yourself relax even more deeply as you continue to focus upon your feet and this time, you raise your right foot a little more out of the water and giving the ankle a slow turn...first this way and then that way. And you do the same movements with your other foot and before you are fully aware of your intent, you have once again brought your left foot forward while your hand is simultaneously reaching out towards it. You touch your ankle gently and lovingly and then you raise both your legs straight up and out of the water and while turning your ankles in gentle circles you look right at them and say quietly, "Thank you, Ankles!"

Next, you bring your hands to each calf one at a time and you massage each one deeply; first on the back calf muscle area and then gently on the front of each of your shins. You marvel at the strength and beauty of your legs and the steam that is rising off of them. And while noticing this and thinking about how important your ankles and calves are to your everyday enjoyment of life you say quietly, "Thank you, Calves!" You notice you are enjoying this attention to self and watching the water streaming down each leg so much, that you feel quite pleasant right now.

Next, you touch your knees, both on the front and back while you think about how important these joints are; how valuable and amazing they really are in the function of your daily life and you quietly thank your knees.

Then you seem to notice your hands in a new way and you take one hand and massage the other, each finger and each palm and you can feel the tingling power of your own touch. Then you think of all the incredible gifts your hands give you and all of the important tasks they carry out daily and you say quietly, while looking at your hands, "Thank you!"

Then you do the same, continuing with each wrist, then each

forearm, then each elbow joint and then your biceps and triceps, thanking them one after the other after taking a moment to recognize each of their special functions. You are becoming more aware of how good this exercise is making you feel, so appreciative of yourself and so aware and so loving. You *like* this.

Now you find yourself rising up out of the tub. You are a beautiful, steaming creation of God. And you think about your upper thighs and then you bend slightly forward to grasp one upper thigh and you give yourself a deep massage on each thigh as you think about all your thighs do for you and then you thank them, too. You next pay attention to your tummy and your chest area, while thinking loving and thankful thoughts for each part of your body and all that it does for you each and every day, each and every moment, often without any conscious thought on your part at all.

You give your buttocks a good jiggle and a rub while you wiggle a little and lovingly think of all that it has done for you, and you quietly thank it. Then you move up your back, thinking of your spine and then your shoulders, touching them, noticing them while you are thanking them.

Finally you reach your neck...your wonderful, sturdy, flexible neck. You thank it and then move your hands to your face, and you notice each feature and each sense: your mouth and its sense of taste, your nose and your sense of smell, your eyes and your sense of sight, your ears and your sense of hearing and you thank each of these features individually and with an acute awareness of their value.

Now you rub your head lightly all over as you thank your scalp and head for all that they do and then when you are done, you let out a big sigh and you let yourself sit back down, sliding into the tub, where the warm water once again envelopes you. This time, not only do you feel relaxed, you feel strangely alive and refreshed, yet deeply peaceful at the same time. You know that somehow, your attention on yourself like this has promoted your own well being and maybe even healing. You are keenly aware of the organ of your skin and all that is good about yourself, all that is healthy, and all that is working just right.

You are filled with a sense of well being and you know that these positive feelings about yourself can do nothing but multiply and you feel gratitude for possessing such an organic system that responds so well to attention, intent and touch. You let out a big sigh and rest back on your pillow, letting your eyes wander once again to the beautiful view.

Now allow yourself to rest for a moment or a while in this state of thankfulness. After returning from this Full Body Thank You guided mediation, you will continue to carry these memories of appreciation and gratitude for yourself and your body...in each and every cell of your being.

Slowly direct your attention to the present moment and bring your awareness back to the now. Feel confident that you have done a good and kind thing for yourself and let a smile stay on your face or deep within you from the experience of this meditation.

Your awareness of all that is good within your body has been increased and you may find yourself doing this exercise on your own, now that you have experienced this process.

The Beach Walk

by Carole Fawcett

As you breathe out tension and breathe in soothing calmness and serenity, see yourself walking on a long, white, sandy beach. It is a breathtakingly beautiful beach and you can see this because you are floating, hovering above the physical "you" that is meandering slowly along the beach, appearing to be deep in thought. You feel the love and calmness waft down from the heavens and wrap around the "you" that is sauntering along the white sands of the seashore. You feel awash with calmness and tranquility.

It is a safe feeling. You feel enveloped in the soothing and healing power of trust, safety and unconditional love. It represents your love for yourself. It feels powerful and you have the knowledge that anything is achievable in this lifetime. You are deeply relaxed and feel safe.

As you feel yourself walking in the sand, you find that you are blending into the other self, becoming one and forming a union of admiration for you and what you have accomplished on your life's journey so far. The emotional, the physical and the spiritual have become one within you.

As you continue to walk along the shore, you are aware of the silky sand caressing your toes and with the occasional tiny wave washing over your feet, you feel as though you are in the womb of Mother Earth...a cocoon of warmth, with only love and peace in your being....your physical, emotional and spiritual being.

You are in awe of this special place of safety, love and total acceptance. It is unconditional and nothing will ever change that.

In the distance, at the end of the sandy beach are large rocks. One rock appears to have the shape of an angel. For some reason, you feel like you know this entity very well. You are not concerned at all, in fact, you want to hurry to reach her. So, you start to skip and almost run along the beach in eager anticipation...feeling the breeze massaging your body as you do.

Finally, you reach her. She is not well defined; she is somewhat of a blur in your vision... veils of thin, white linen billow around her in an ethereal manner...and yet...she seems real and present.

You ask her what her name is and the wind whispers it to you.

Your emotions surge with joyfulness and again the wind whispers...*"All is well in your world and happiness is acknowledging the moment and allowing your being to fill up with gratitude for what is."*

Take a moment now to feel the gratitude fill your body. Allow it to scan your entire body, stopping where healing energy is required. Gratitude heals. Forgiveness heals.

The power of gratitude has imbued your cells with strong and healthy energy. You are full of wonder at this feeling and gratitude washes over your body again and again.

The angel begins to fade and you quickly thank her for sharing her wisdom...within minutes the vision of her has faded and you are left feeling empowered as you walk along the beach...back the way you came.

You stop and look back once again, seeing the rock formation. It is a beautiful rock that has been carved by the sea waters washing against it since the beginning of time. Part of it appears to take the form of an angel's wing.

Once again, you feel the loving calm and peace wash over you. It feels *so* good.

You feel the connection to Mother Earth, to the sea, to the natural rhythm of nature and to all the living beings that share this planet.

You have unified your energies and now you are physically, emotionally and spiritually one within yourself.

Take a moment and enjoy this realization.

Relaxation in Two Parts

by Paula Reynolds

And now...As you drift deeper and deeper down ...Breathing in and out...In and out...Exhaling deeply ...Further and further down you go...You feel a sense of peacefulness you've never experienced before...It wraps around you in a blanket of comfort and you feel all stresses slowly drifting away...So far away that they are like distant memories that no longer have any meaning...You sink into the chair and feel it supporting all of your weight...You focus on the top of your head as it gets heavier and heavier, supported by the chair...You continue to breathe deeply and fully...In and out...In and out...This feeling now moves into your eyes as the lids grow heavier and heavier...You can no longer open your eyes...They are tightly shut and this is comforting to you...Going deeper and deeper still...Breathing deeply...Now the feeling moves into your jaw as it drops open slightly and you exhale through your mouth...Very deeply...Breathing in and out...And letting this beautiful feeling flood over you...It now moves into your shoulders as they become very heavy and relaxed...There is no tension in them at all...

You are experiencing a wave of extreme peace and relaxation that is washing over you as you drift deeper and deeper down...It now continues down through your back and chest...You are feeling so peaceful and pleasantly heavy in your blanket of comfort...Your entire spine is loose and relaxed...The chair supports you as you feel this extreme peace and relaxation...Enjoy the support and let your body continue to go limp and heavy as this relaxation moves through your stomach and into your hips...You feel your hips grow heavier and heavier as all stresses drift away...Breathing in and out...In and out...Going deeper and deeper with every breath...Feeling the peaceful heaviness of your body and the support of the chair...Focus on this support and the sound of my voice as you breathe deeply...In and out...Now this peaceful heaviness is moving into your legs...Feel your legs being supported...Feel how heavy they are now...Let the chair support their weight as the weight of the world is lifted from you...Breathing deeply...In and out...Drifting deeper and deeper...Deeper and deeper down...Your legs are relaxing all the way from your hips to your ankles...A beautiful relaxation that moves down your legs in a peaceful heaviness...Breathing in and out...And allowing your body to relax fully as it is supported by the chair...Drifting deeper and deeper down...Deeper and deeper down...Now you feel the heaviness of your feet as the peaceful heaviness drifts down into them...You feel the stresses drifting away and you are now fully rooted in a beautiful relaxation that completely envelopes you in a comforting, peaceful blanket...Just enjoy this feeling of complete relaxation and peaceful heaviness...Know that you can come back to this place anytime you choose...You have the control and the power to recreate this feeling anytime that is right and perfect for you...You just breathe deeply and imagine the heaviness moving from the top of your head all the way down to your feet...And let go of everything...You are powerful and in control...You can relax anytime that is right and perfect for you...And in the way that is right and perfect for you...Anytime and anywhere and in any way that is perfect for you...

And now that you are fully relaxed and peaceful, I want you to visualize or imagine that you are standing at the edge of a prairie grassland...It is a beautiful day with bright blue skies and some big, white, fluffy clouds...There is a light wind that helps to cool you off in the heat of the day...You feel totally comfortable and relaxed as you look across this landscape with its endless miles in front of you...You breathe in and out and feel more and more relaxed with each breath...You are alone and safe in this big landscape and this brings you more peace and relaxation...You see the rolling flatness of the land and the short brown and green grasses that gently wave in the wind...You see the birds as they dip and float in the sky...You hear their songs and this music takes you even deeper into relaxation...You can feel yourself breathing deeply...In and out...In and out...And all cares and stresses float away as all your senses take in the scene before you...You now find a gentle path and start to walk through the landscape, feeling the strength of your body and finding a quiet comfort in this...You feel the gentle dips and rises in the path as you slowly make your way down it, enjoying the feeling of being in the present...Enjoying the strength of your body and mind...

Your mind is focused on this moment and all thoughts and concerns of another time are gone...Your shoes are comfortable and support you...Your clothing is perfectly suited to this climate...The sun and wind and temperature are at the perfect setting for you...There is no discomfort or stress at all...You breathe in and out...In and out...Inhaling deeply...And exhaling deeply...Follow the path and enjoy the peacefulness of just being in the moment...You feel the glorious sun on your face with all its healing powers...All around you as you pass are tiny flowers of various brilliant colors...There are some small bushes that wave gently in the breeze...And when you want shade there are some large, beautiful trees to pause under...You can pick one to sit under or just wander around and enjoy the shade...If you want you can give one of these trees a hug and feel its strength that is much like your own...

All decisions you make are easy and simple...You follow your heart and instinctively know what is best for you...Everything you do is in your best interest and feels right and perfect for you...Everything...And you continue to breathe in and out deeply...Going deeper and deeper into relaxation with each breath...There is nowhere else you want to be right now...And this feels absolutely perfect for you...Everything is perfect for you...And you know that you can come back to this place anytime you choose...You are in control and you are powerful...You create your life...You can create the life that you want and live it in the way that you want... Peacefulness is yours and you now understand this and fully feel it...You are ready to create this peacefulness in your life...You are ready to take control of your life...And now, with these thoughts in your mind and these feelings in your heart, you are ready to start walking back to the edge of the prairie grassland...You are ready to come back to your life and make it peaceful and positive...You are in control and you know what you want out of life...You are ready to create the life that is right and perfect for you...You are in control and you will create this life...And so it is.

Turn Up the Heat in Digestion, Metabolism and Energy

by Kit Muehlman

A Meditation/Induction with Inner Fire Focus using the map of the Yoga Koshas or layers of being.

This is a meditation using the element of Fire, an element of intensity, transformation, and creativity. Our bodies naturally produce heat as we burn food and turn matter into energy. We produce so much internal heat that we're most comfortable in external environments 20 to 30 degrees cooler than our internal temperature. The element of fire combines with our desires to fuel our intentions. We add fire to our intentions to inspire actions, and our actions shape our lives.

Begin by sitting or lying down. If you're warm, you can take off your shoes, or if you think you might cool down, a light blanket can be useful. Find a position that allows you to relax your muscles and be comfortably warm.

(*Physical Body*) Take a deep breath, hold it in for a moment, and let it go whenever you're ready, and then let your breath flow naturally, an easy inhale...and soft exhale. If you like, you can close your eyes to make it easier to turn inward. As you watch your breathing...you'll notice cool air flowing into your nostrils...and warm air flowing out ...your body releases heat through breathing...and through your skin...

Now bring your attention to the solar plexus, the space above your navel...deep in the center of your body. This is the center of digestion, where your body burns the food you eat, where the digestive fire resides, transforming food into

42

energy. Allow your attention to hover around your abdomen...Breathe deeply into your abdomen to invite a clean steady digestion.

You may be aware of the heat radiating from the warm core of your body through your skin. Allow the heat in your body to relax you...let the outer layer of your body soften ...becoming more and more aware of what you're experiencing internally...letting your attention move inward...as you notice places where you might be able to relax even more...

(*Energetic Body*) As you watch your breath...you can call to mind the myriad chemical combustions taking place at the cellular level...sparks of electricity in the muscles, nerves, and brain...As long as you breathe, this energy is unstoppable...

You are a portable power plant, fueled by the food you eat and the oxygen you breathe...even your experiences feed into your power...as your body responds...every moment, to your experiences...with chemicals such as adrenaline, cortisol, and serotonin...Watch the movement of your breath...the oxygen fanning the blue flame of your power...slowly and steadily...unhurried, unforced.

(*Mental/Emotional Body*) Even while you rest...your consciousness keeps firing thoughts...like it's cleaning out and burning up old to-do lists...powering you forward in time and space...powering you onward through life. Your mind sifting through deep desires...examining motivations and intentions...Your breath fans the flames of your power, tempering and strengthening your will...spontaneously and naturally, without forcing.

(*Inner Wisdom Body*) And isn't it interesting to rest and watch, knowing your inner thermostats are automatically and spontaneously regulating the inner fires... spontaneously organizing thoughts, without even trying...

(*Bliss Body*) Drifting down, deeper and deeper down, to the place before thoughts begin...resting in the space between breaths...a place where everything just is...alive and pulsing...not trying to make anything happen...just noticing your experience, the experience of breathing...not trying to make your breath go any particular way...making room for what's happening, with kindness and curiosity...Let any sensations float in softness and openness...Thoughts may come and go, evaluating, remembering...it doesn't matter, just noticing.

In a few moments, I'm going to ask you to come back to full wakefulness and consensus reality, so you can take some time now to experience the power of your breath...the power inside you that's innate, unforced...the essence of creative impulse...You can call on this power by slowing down, watching your breath...and listening without trying to make anything happen...listening to the space between breaths...patiently...breathing softly on the flame of aliveness...feeling the cool air on the inhale...the warmth of the exhale...knowing that when you come back into wakeful awareness, your mind will feel clearer, the air will feel fresher, and life will feel a little easier...Your activities will flow with a delightful creative power, powered by fires deep within, and the steady fuel of your breath.

Now invite a deeper breath into your lungs, let the oxygen flow to your arms and legs fingers and toes, stretch, and when you're ready, you can open your eyes.

Journey to Calmness

by Jackie Foskett

This journey to calmness provides a special time for you to simple let go and delight in the feelings of peacefulness, calmness, serenity and joy.

Each time you listen to this, you continue to build your reservoir, your fund of inner calm. This inner calm fund represents your investment in you and the return is your immediate access to your health and well being.

Simply find a comfortable place to sit or lie down. This is your quiet time now. This is your journey.

Begin now by bringing your attention to your breath...that's right, simply breathe in and out at your normal pace...as you do...notice how your breath feels in your nasal passages as you inhale, and how it feels as you exhale out either through your nose or through your mouth...whatever is most comfortable for you now...simply observe the breath...good.

Notice how your abdomen rises and falls with each and every inhale and then exhale...

Inhaling easily...exhaling...easily...good.

Now, when you are ready...allow yourself to take a very deep breath in...way down into your abdomen...and then slowly exhale out...Each and every breath brings in life giving oxygen that circulates around and begins to soften all the muscles in your body...every cell...way down deep into the cellular level...and as you exhale...you allow any tension to be released...and you sink deeper into relaxation...

letting go...relaxing...releasing...going within now...allowing your breath to breathe you into relaxation now...

As you breathe yourself into relaxation with each and every breath...your imagination becomes more fluid...and you can easily imagine now...that as the thoughts that naturally come into your mind...can either be simple background sound...or you might imagine a soft gentle breeze clearing them out as they come in...

And, if you choose to clear them out with a soft gentle breeze...you can create a container to your side that captures those thoughts so that, in the event you would like them back later, you can simply retrieve them from the container. But for now...either allow them to go into the container or have them be background sound, either way...there is no need to give them your attention now...this is your time to let go... relax and go on a special journey in your mind and imagination.

That's right...

Now, as you continue to breathe yourself into relaxation, with that wonderful relaxing oxygen that you are receiving, and then release with every exhale...your imagination continues to become more fluid, as your conscious mind begins to slow down...and that's a good thing right now...slowing down...as you deserve to slow down and allow relaxation to permeate your entire body...

Imagine now...a warm soothing light surrounding your entire body now...this light is a color that you find very soothing. As it surrounds your entire body, it allows you to feel very warm, safe, comfortable and protected.

As you feel warm, comfortable, safe and protected, it is that much easier for you to simply let go, release and go within, into that place within you that knows how to feel calm, at peace and relaxed.

Continuing now to drift down into a very comfortable state of relaxation with each and every breath you take...

Notice the support beneath you...and as you exhale...allowing yourself to simply sink down into that support...knowing you are fully supported now...

In a moment, I'm going to count down from 10-1, each descending number as well as the sound of my voice will allow you to let go more and more. And you may even be curious and you may wonder, today, just how deep you can go as you hear each number and you may experience a deeper level of relaxation...inner focus...deep safe hypnosis...than you've ever experienced before...as you focus on my voice and then each number...now...

10, letting go, into your own inner essence...9...releasing more now...8...it feels good to let go...as you drift down to 7...releasing more and more now as you easily go down to 6....letting go...down to 5...relaxing down 4...this is your special time...as you continue to easily release as you drift down still deeper within...still deeper down to 3......deeper still... down 2...deep deep relaxation...and now...go way down deeper...all the way down to 1......good!

And now, as you take another breath deep down into your abdomen, you sink still deeper down...way, way down into a deep pleasant state of relaxation and inner focus...feeling so safe...and comfortable...in this wonderful deep hypnotic state...

As you drift down more and more...your imagination becomes ever more fluid now...as you imagine...a beautiful place in nature, perhaps a place you've been before, or perhaps a place you've longed to go to, or perhaps simply a place you create right now in your mind and imagination. This is a place where you can be alone and yet never feel lonely...a place where you feel very safe and very secure...a place where you are at one with all there is...

Experience being there fully now...as you notice the colors you see in your beautiful place in nature...notice the feel of the temperature of the air on your skin...notice if there are any aromas you can smell here in this beautiful place in nature...and notice...if there are any sounds you can hear...or perhaps...all you hear is the sound of silence...

And notice, especially now...how very calm, peaceful and serene you feel being here in this beautiful place in nature. Enjoy being here completely now.

As you continue enjoying this experience...you become aware there is a path that looks very inviting. It's surrounded by such beautiful flowers and greenery. It's nice and wide to comfortably walk down.

Imagine yourself walking down this path now, feeling very comfortable and in awe of such beauty along the way.

You are very much present to all that is here along this special path...as it meanders gently down...and you continue following it easily down...trusting you are on the right path for you...

You keep noticing all the beauty along this path and it fills you with such deep appreciation.

Mother Nature in her most creative expression...and you are experiencing the incredibleness of it all...feeling good, feeling at one with Mother Earth...as you continue walking down this safe beautiful path.

As you continue walking down, you become aware of the sound of a stream...its gentle, calm, downward flow of water...getting closer...now...as you continue going down this path...and then it appears...and you watch how it flows so easily over twigs, rocks...continuing to flow with ease..and you notice, too how soothing it is to simply observe its flow...

You see some leaves floating on by and they glide downstream with ease...you can easily imagine those leaves are like any worries, any persistent thoughts that you had before you came on this journey...and you imagine those worries, thoughts, concerns are simply floating away on those leaves...gently easily...floating away...

Any of those thoughts you had before...that are really important...will naturally be collected somewhere downstream where you can gather them up...when you need them...when it is appropriate for you to attend to them...but for now...this is your special place and your special time...everything has its time...and this is your time for relaxing and letting go.

For now...you just let them go...and you continue walking down this path now...with ease and comfort and a new sense of awe...as you explore...new ways of being...so calm, so serene...so at one with all of Nature...it feels so good...everything flows...just like the stream...easily...no struggle here...it's all flowing smoothly...

The path continues to meander around so gracefully and you easily follow it...there is an inner knowingness now...that tells you...this is very real...this is good...this is the right path to be on now...

You are aware of the warm rays of the sunshine filtering through the greenery as you walk along...giving you the exact right lighting...soft...comfortable...warm...and you marvel at how good that feels...

As you are marveling at how good you feel, you notice up ahead that the stream has found its way into a lovely pool of water.

This pool is surrounded by natural rocks and soft ferns and it has an outlet you can see that allows the water to continue flowing...you know this is very clean fresh water here in this pool...it's constantly being refreshed...replenished...restored to its depth...a depth that allows for floating in it...as well as standing...and you wonder...you wonder if you could float in this pool...it's so inviting...you feel drawn to go into this lovely water...and so you decide to feel the temperature of this pool...perhaps with a toe or your hand...ahh...you discover...it's just the right temperature for you to go into...it's warm...it's soothing...it's very comfortable...

You can see to the bottom...it's just the right amount of water for you and you feel so comfortable and safe and know it's perfectly safe to go into this pool of water...

And...so you let yourself go into this pool of water that's being renewed all the time...and it feels so good to simply let go and go in...

It's just the right temperature...it's so refreshing and it's so lovely...it puts an immediate smile on your face...and you find you feel playful....you feel joyous...you are delighted...

You are dipping in and out of this water...having fun...feeling so alive...and good...feeling so relaxed as you play in this pool...it feels so good to let go and play...you are loving it...you are smiling, laughing...and completely enjoying yourself...ahh...

And then you decide to simply lay on your back and float, even if you've never done that before...you know it's something that is perfectly fine for you to do right now...ahh...it's easy...wow...you notice the water is holding

50

you up, with no effort on your part at all...and...you realize...you can completely let go and relax...this is a healing pool...a magical healing pool...

You are thoroughly enjoying yourself in this healing pool...just floating...feeling so good, feeling very, very relaxed...knowing that all is well...all is well...feeling connected to Mother Nature in a whole, new way now...feeling connected to yourself...feeling connected to life...feeling immense love...for Nature...all that is...and for yourself...

You continue floating now...in this very safe and healing place...and...you continue letting go...you know innately that all is well...you now know at a whole, new level...how your own, innate brilliance led you down the wonderful path to this incredibly soothing, healing pool of water...it's so calming...it's so restful...it's so refreshing...

As you look around at the water, you notice how blue it is...just like the blue sky you can see through the trees in this wonderful place in nature...

The color blue resonates throughout your body...allowing you to feel even more calm...in choice...present...being here...enjoying...feeling good...feeling life...feeling so fulfilled and feeling so appreciative of this experience...

You are simply connected in the now...to who you really are...the essence of your pure spirit...This is where you naturally and easily connect to your creativity...your aliveness, your innate brilliance...where you can easily know what's best for you...and so you keep allowing that connection to be present for you...and it feels so good and it feels so natural...and it feels so right for you.

And now you decide...it's time to get up from your heavenly blue pool of water...this water that completely supported you

51

as you let go and trusted in its innate healing abilities...you are choosing to continue moving forward now...having allowed yourself this time of being completely connected to who you really are...

You effortlessly ease out of the pool and you easily dry off...the temperature of the air is just right...and you look at this pool of water that keeps itself renewed with the fresh water coming from the down flowing stream...and you know you will always remember this experience...it is completely in your body...this feeling...this calmness...the serenity you felt...and still feel now...

And you know you can always return here...you can take your walk down your path and come to this healing, relaxing pool and play and then simply float, relax and enjoy the moment...feeling the restoration come into you as you do...feeling the calmness permeate your entire body...feeling that calmness staying with you...as your body soaks it up...yes...you can come back anytime you like, anytime you begin to notice you need renewal...you need some play...you need some calmness and joy...

This is your very own special floating and healing pool...it is within you now...and will continue to be replenished by the down flowing stream which connects you to who you really are...

And when you are ready...find yourself now...continuing your walk along your beautiful path...the path that led you to your own healing place, your own healing pool...the path that will continue to lead you into calmness, restoration, play, and joy...and your innate brilliance...

A Perfect Place

by Vivienne Barker

Following induction and deepener:

I want you to imagine now...You are standing in your perfect place...positive, calm and tranquil...so still and perfect... precious...peaceful and beautiful...This is a place of purpose and caring that is...loving...living...and alive within you.

This perfect place deep within you is a place that has always been there...all along and will always be, just for you alone.

You search for the place as it appears...elusive, yet illuminating...while safely holding all of your positive thoughts and feelings...your most intimate thoughts and feelings...things known only by you and you alone...

In this positive place you can heal yourself...this place that is just for you and you alone...your perfect place....

You are embraced here in a wonderful, healing light...the glow of the colors are in harmony with you and your positive thoughts...

Each ray of light that touches you...caresses you...each and every color that wraps around you...dissolves any negative emotions. Burdens of pain, loneliness and despair...cannot thrive in your perfect place...they depart your perfect place or...they must evolve to survive...pain melts away into resolve, loneliness becomes a lioness, despair turns to hope and with a new, powerful and positive sense of well being...

You now welcome and celebrate the transformation ...feeling relief as those old emotions are transformed and...released...

This perfect place of peace waits for you...this place deep within you...that has eternally waited for you...waited to care for you...love you unconditionally...silent in its acceptance... still in its admiration...its quietly loving contemplation...this place deep within you...This perfect place deep within you is a place that has always been there...all along and will always be...just for you alone.

Gratitude

by Monika Burton

In a consultation with your client, ask about: phobias, fears, allergies to food or animals, eating habits, health issues, and adjust the script accordingly. Find out about your client's gifts and skills and what they enjoy doing. Explain the principle behind; "When you change the way you look at things, the things you look at change".

Ask the client for permission to give them a small piece of fruit during the session. (I like using a strawberry or a raspberry, something that will dissolve easily).

Close your eyes... get yourself in a nice comfortable position...Take a deep breath in and exhale...getting ready for deep relaxation...just allow your body to relax...as you are breathing in and out...relaxing more and more with each breath you take. Your breath is such a powerful tool...you notice how easy it is for you to relax...with each breath in and each exhalation...relaxing your body, relaxing your mind, breathe in...your body is relaxing even more and more...with each breath...relaxing even deeper and deeper.

Noticing how your body is becoming heavier and heavier...you can almost feel your body sinking into the chair/bed...Your head is sinking into the pillow (chair)...As you are starting to relax...so nicely...so deeply... deeper...and deeper into relaxation. This time is just for you...allowing yourself to relax deeply...it feels so good to relax mentally...more and more...nothing to think about right now...nothing to worry about...That's right...

Thoughts can be thought...but you may just imagine your

thoughts floating away...let them pass by....for now....let them just float away...there's nothing, nothing of importance for you to do right now...except to relax...physically and mentally...more ...and more...drifting deeper and deeper...As you continue to relax...going deeper and deeper ...it's easier it is for you to listen and to follow the sound of my voice...relaxing so nicely...noticing now how your body is becoming heavier and heavier...the deeper into relaxation you go. And the deeper you go...the better you feel.

I may ask you to speak to me or to show me a sign during this session...this will not disturb you in any way...If you speak, the sound of your voice will take you deeper and deeper into a beautiful hypnotic state...so that as you speak, with every sound of your voice or by giving me a sign...you will drift deeper and deeper into trance. Any sounds outside or inside of the room...will not affect you or disturb you in any way...in fact, these sounds will help you and guide you to be more and more relaxed. During the hypnosis, I will come closer to you and at one point I will offer you a piece of fruit, placing it on top of your tongue...and that will allow you to stay in a deep state of relaxation...the smell, the taste and the feeling of the fruit will take you even deeper and deeper...just as my voice...and the music...will take you deeper and deeper into hypnosis.

Now imagine in your mind's eye or sense that you are at a place where you feel safe... some place where you feel protected and at peace. Maybe it is a place you have visited before, a place where you like to go and relax or you can just create such a peaceful place in your mind, with your imagination...Go to that space now. Imagine or sense the feeling of being here...it feels so good, so safe...such a great place to be...breathe in...are there any scents? Maybe you can hear sounds...perhaps it is warm there...sunny, and you can feel the warmth on your skin...or a gentle breeze...Feeling free, safe and relaxed. Allow yourself to observe the surroundings...look around...enjoy it...Wherever you are... enjoy the safety and the comfort of this place.

Now, in this beautiful, safe place...find a comfortable place to rest...allow yourself to feel comfortable...wherever you are...make yourself comfortable...enjoy...that's right...

And now I want you to imagine a bright white light or any other color you choose...this light is coming down from above your head, entering your body. It is a powerful, healing light ...feel its relaxing energy spreading through your entire body...that's right...and you feel so good...

This light is coming from above, spreading the energy to every single cell, and the space between the cells, calming your nervous system, flowing through your back, sliding around your spine...and into each vertebra...as it is becoming perfectly aligned, filling your body with healing energy... energizing...rejuvenating...healing...strengthening... visualize it, feel it, sense it...

Send this energy into your spine, into your joints, your bones, your muscles and tendons...from the top of your head to the bottom of your feet...all the way to your toes...just relaxing you...healing you.

Any tensions just melt away...as you are relaxing, healing, energizing...this healing light...this healing energy is flowing so nicely through your body...Your body is relaxing so beautifully now...deeply...that's right...You can take some time now to enjoy it, to scan the body...feeling the power of the healing light...it feels so good...

(This can be augmented with full body relaxation, starting with the top of the head)

Ask for permission and give your client a very small piece of fruit. Hold the fruit (strawberry or raspberry) in front of the clients nose .. or ask them to imagine it...in front of their nose .. so they can smell it .. or sense its scent. And then, put it in their mouth.

In a moment, I will move closer to you and hold a piece of *(name of the fruit)* in front of you...allowing you to enjoy the smell of this fruit...and now I am going to gently place this *(raspberry)* on top of your tongue...Allow it to melt...feel the juice in your mouth... enjoy the taste and the tartness...or the subtle sweetness on top of your tongue..You can taste it melting in your mouth...And when you swallow it you can imagine or feel it becoming part of your body...Your body is taking in all the nutrients and all the vitamins ...transforming it into energy...into life force...That's right...enjoy the taste, appreciate the nutrients, appreciate your ability to enjoy all the sweetness or sometimes the bitterness...It is such a gift that you have...the ability to eat (healthy, delicious) food...it is a gift to have access to all this amazing, fresh, good quality food...

And as you feel the taste or the aftertaste in your mouth...or on your tongue...the feeling of gratitude is filling you...for all of the food...which allows you to be strong and healthy ...food which your body is turning into energy...allowing you to move, to exercise, to stretch, to be strong, to dance, to sing...so that you can walk...the wonderful gift: the ability to go for a beautiful walk, to enjoy the scenery around you...to hike and to explore...you can go places...

You are grateful for all your abilities to do all of these things...to be able to see, to taste, to touch and observe...Being able to smell the sweetness of a flower or the freshness of a tree...Such a simple thing as the ability to taste the sweetness of the fruit or the smell of fruit...The abilities to be able to do the things you love to do, being able to hear sounds... perhaps sounds of beautiful music ...or sounds of nature...how great it feels to become lost in the sound of the music or the sound of the ocean...and the next time you are in nature..or even just at home, you take a few moments from time to time, to stop and allow the feelings of gratitude for all the gifts you have, to be able to be who you are, where you are right now...

Allow yourself to appreciate these feelings of gratitude for all the gifts you have...*(list here your client's gifts and skills)*...You are enjoying the feelings of gratitude for all of these wonderful gifts and talents that you have...

And now I want you to imagine in your mind's eye how nice it feels to be hugged or to hug someone very special...or how it feels to hold a baby...how does it feel to be in their presence...or perhaps how it feels to hold and hug an animal you love. Feeling the love...it feels so good...it is so beautiful to be in a presence of someone or something you love...

And now I would like you to remember the time or the situation when you have helped someone or when you did something nice for somebody...you are remembering the feeling... allowing yourself to feel it now...the feeling of giving...the feeling of sharing...the feeling of being appreciated...It is such a wonderful gift...Imagine how good it feels to be able to do something nice for someone else. Remember how good it feels... tp give yourself a gift and do something nice for another person...often...Knowing something as little as a nice smile or just saying something nice to someone is a gift...

You can take a deep breath now...soaking in all these feelings of gratitude for all the senses, for the (beautiful, strong, healthy) body you have...enjoying the gifts of being able to share your energy with others...and appreciation for others who share their energy with you...gratitude for all of your friends and all the beautiful people and others who are coming into your life, teaching you, guiding you, protecting you.

Beginning now, you are very aware of the power of your choice. The choice you have to look at things...Remembering "when you change the way you look at things, the things you look at change"...Knowing and standing in your power, creating your new life, filled with happiness and joy...Your ability to look at things in a positive way...attracting positive energy into your life...That's right. *(add other suggestions suitable for your client)*

Create an anchor: Now, listen carefully...you will be able to remember and recreate this amazing feeling of gratitude, the feeling of empowerment, confidence and gratitude with ...your special smile, and every time you...have this special smile, you will feel all that energy flowing into your body, reflecting into your body posture, increasing your confidence, feeling good. Imagine how it feels to stand in your power, in your confidence, in your gratitude. It feels so good.

Unconscious Ocean

by Jocelyn L.H. Jensen

One thing that has really annoyed me over the years amid hypnotic induction techniques, is the "breathe in through the nose and out through the mouth" instruction. Anyone who has been subjected to this breathing technique can feel just how unnatural it really is; yet it is the standard beginning for many mainstream inductions of hypnosis.

Today, let's try something much more natural...something I actually learned in Hatha Yoga...abdominal, or "belly breathing". I will guide you through it, as it may not feel natural at first. The reason for that is in abdominal breathing, you have no choice...you must be AWARE of the movements of your body and organs as you breathe, and also you must be aware of the movement of the air on its passage into and out of your body. You will find that this mode of aware breathing is much more conducive to the experience of hypnotic trance.

To begin this process, place your dominant hand comfortably on your stomach, and just continue to listen to the sound of my voice. Follow my instructions carefully, and simply notice the feelings that develop.

We begin now. Breathe in through your nose. Imagine your breath as a visible stream traveling up through your nostrils, into your windpipe, and down to the very bottom of your lungs as you inhale deeply. At the same time as you do this, become aware of how your belly expands under your hand. Fill your lungs completely and at the completion of the

61

inhalation, pause for just a second, and then exhale just as completely as you inhaled. Feel the breath as it leaves your lungs, returns through your windpipe, and exits your nostrils. Note that as you exhale, your belly naturally contracts, all by itself.

Does the air have a color as you inhale, and does that color change on the exhale? If so, this is fine, and if not it is also fine. Allow this abdominal expansion and contraction cycle to find its own comfortable and natural rhythm as you continue to listen.

As you focus and concentrate...and listen, you may find that your mind has a tendency to wander back and forth...back and forth...from my words...to your breathing...from your breathing...to my words. A secondary rhythm... complementary to the pace of your breath.

Focus...concentrate...listen...wander...breath to words... words to breath...air to Voice...Voice to Air. The two rhythms pace each other...then lead each other...your mind weaving in and out of them...back and forth of them...betwixt and between them. Soon you find...paying attention to your breathing is...no longer important...it just continues on its own...deeply in...and completely out...deeply in...and completely out.

And since that deep belly breath is now automatic...that means that your unconscious mind...has caught the gist...the core of meaning...of what I wanted. Your automatic breathing...has freed your mind...to give its attention to my words...fully and completely.

Focusing now on the sound of my voice...more than on the words I speak. Find that your focus is narrowing...more and more aware of my voice...less and less aware of the world. Your conscious mind, enjoying the comfort you feel now...even as your unconscious mind begins...to know curiosity...to wonder...what it would be like to allow...the experience...of a deep and comfortable hypnotic state.

Now your unconscious mind...may want to go very deeply into hypnosis...while your conscious mind...may prefer a lighter state. But as in the state of trance, the unconscious is in the driver's seat, what the conscious mind wants, simply doesn't matter. The sound of my voice calls out to your unconscious...and the conscious mind...simply...submerges ...now.

And you feel absolutely wonderful...as you drift, float and dream...on the currents of my words. My voice...a broad but gently flowing river...and you know...what the destination ...of all rivers is...the River of Dreams...flows down to the Sea of Dreams...gently buoyant...full of promise.

The vast Ocean...of the Unconscious...bottomless ...limitless...a Wellspring Resource...holding all one needs... to live...to grow...to change...to become.

What will you become today? With boundaries gone, how far will you travel? With limits removed...How much will you grow? All you need...every ingredient...contained here... in your Unconscious Ocean. You imagine now...your positive outcome...even as...hypnosis goes deeper.

Hypnosis goes deeper...currents waft you...drifting and dreaming...in your Unconscious Ocean...safely buoyed... within yourself...as the dream...grows more profound. Unconscious mind...researches ways...researches means...of comfort...of depth...of growth...of change.

Change is...the Universal Constant...without change...inertia takes over. Inertia is...the Great Remover...of the Creative ...of the New. Inertia wants...to keep things static; but in Life, all must move...all must grow. As Life grows...Life finds ways...to create the betterment, of all that lives.

Create Your best Life...create your True Dream...see and feel that deep dream now...float to the surface of your Unconscious Ocean...ready to be...netted and taken.

Take that Dream onboard your Mind-Boat...pour its fuel...into your Soul-engine. Newly fuelled, and newly charted...set the course...weigh the anchor. Travelling the length...plumbing the depths...charting the breadth...of the Unconscious Ocean...enjoy the journey of your newly fuelled Life.

Become once more...aware of your breathing...see and feel it slowly changing...from deep to shallower, from sleep to awake...your mind emerges...from this journey. The count now brings you, to where you started...relaxed, alert...and ready to LIVE.

From 1 to 10...and back you come now...return to awareness...loving life. 1...2...3...4...5...noticing the room around you...6...7...aware of new determination and life-purpose...6...5...half asleep again...4...feeling so good...3... and you...2...go all the way...1...back down and deep...0 ...nowwww.

From 1 to 10...and back you come now...return to awareness...loving life...Feeling the energy of the Universe itself...filling you up from top to toe. You are now so full of Life...you won't be able to help but grow!

Focus On "The Now"

By: Carole Fawcett

This helps to stop the "Monkey Mind" (Thoughts like monkeys that swing from neuron to neuron, interfering with a sense of peace or disrupting sleep...keeping one in a continual state of worry, etc.)

I would like you to focus on this moment as you hear my voice. Focus on my voice, the present, how your body feels on the couch/recliner, how warm you feel...the soothing sounds in the room.

Take a moment to focus on these things. Do not allow any other thoughts to enter your mind. Keep focused on this very moment. Be mindful with your thoughts. You *can* do this because *you* are in charge of your mind and your thoughts. You do not need to rent space to any thoughts in your head that do not create positive, joyful and peaceful results. You are in charge of that space.

Focus...stay focused on the relaxation, my voice, the fountain, the music...focus on how relaxed you feel right now. No worries from yesterday and what did happen, no worries about the future and what 'might' happen. Just focused on right now...nothing else... right now. Concentrate and do not allow your mind to go anywhere except where you want it to go.

Rein in your thoughts...keep them mindful on what is happening now...do not allow other thoughts to creep in. If something continues to creep in, create a container in your mind. You have the creativity and the ability to design a special container...with a lid... decorating it as you wish.

Take a moment and do that now.

So, now when you have thoughts about the past or the future that keep interfering with your relaxation or your quality of life, put them into your beautiful container, close the lid and lock it. Put the key in a safe place in your mind. Only you can open this and only when you choose to do so.

Now, creating a whiteboard in your mind's eye, pick up the marker on the ledge of the whiteboard...making it any colour you like. There are several markers on the ledge and they are all different colours.

With the first marker, write in capital letters on the whiteboard: I AM LIVING IN THE NOW. (or *THIS MOMENT*) Write it in the middle of the whiteboard...then erase it. Next, write it on the left side of the whiteboard, one word under the other...then erase it. Next, write it on the bottom of the whiteboard...then erase it. Next, write it diagonally across the whiteboard...then erase it.

Now, write these words:

I FEEL SAFE AND SECURE IN MY RELATIONSHIPS (*or: I FEEL SAFE AND SECURE WHEN I FLY, GO UP A LADDER, DRIVE THE CAR, etc.*)

Using the different coloured markers, write those words in several places on the white board, leaving them on the board...in the middle, on the sides, at the bottom, at the top.

You are doing extremely well.

66

If you need to stop and put any interfering thoughts into your container, let me know by lifting the fore finger of your right hand...at any time during this session. I will stop and allow you time to do that. When you are finished putting things into your container, you will simply lift the thumb of your right hand to let me know.

So relaxed, so content, so tranquil and serene...you are feeling *smooth* and calm. Continue to concentrate on this moment only. Focus and do not allow any other thoughts to enter your mind.

You can train your brain to live in the moment, not to future-think and worry about what 'might be"...staying focused instead on 'what is'.

Know that you can practice this at home, just prior to going to sleep at night, or using it as a meditation during the day.

You are in charge of your thoughts and when you choose to have them. You will not allow self-limiting beliefs to enter your mind and if they do sneak in, you will catch them with a mind net, put them into your container and lock them up.

You are learning how to live in the now and focus on the good that is happening in your life.

You will be successful with this.

Pregnancy Script

by Leta Heuer

A gentle guided relaxation and breath work process to prepare for childbirth.

Find yourself a comfortable spot and give yourself permission to take time to relax and let go of your daily distractions...giving yourself and your baby that all important together time. Gently let your eyelids meet, welcome that serene feeling that comes by simply allowing all of the muscles in and around your eyes to release and relax. Notice that warm feeling that waves over your body as those muscles relax.

I would like you to take a deep breath...let it out...relaxing your thoughts, relaxing your body...very good. Allow your body to relax. Allow your thoughts to relax. Relax, relax and go deeper.

Next, I am going to count to ten; and with every number I count, I would like you to take a deep breath and each time I say the word exhale simply allow the breath to rush from your body and relax. Again, with every number that I count, I take a deep breath; when you hear the word "exhale" simply let go, relax and allow the breath to leave your body.

(*Proceed to count with each deep breath in and exhale*)

Good...very good...now continue to breath at the perfect pace for your body, find your rhythm, breath and exhale to your rhythm...

Please direct your attention to your toes. Turn your attention toward the tips of your toes. Focus, focus your attention on the very tips of those toes. I would like you to tighten the muscles in your toes. Tighten the muscles in your feet and in your toes in whatever manner you chose hold them very, very tight...hold them...and release, relax them. Good, so very good. Now I would like you to tighten the muscles in your legs, in your calves all the way up your thighs tighten them...hold them...and relax...relax. Very good.

Now gently tighten the muscles in your back and core hold them...and relax...let go. Breathe. Now tighten the muscles in your hands and in your fingers...tighten hold them very, very tightly...hold them...and relax. Now the muscles in your arms ...the forearms, those muscles in your upper arms make them very tight , very, very tightly...hold them...and relax... good, very good. Just let them go limp.

Now very importantly...tense up those shoulder muscles...go ahead, tighten them up in the shoulders and the neck, then release...release and completely relax. Feel the warmth that flows through your body...allow it to move up to your face and tighten all those facial muscles. Tighten them all, around the eyes, the ears the jaw, hold them...tighten them and release, relax simply let go, let all those little muscles completely relax. You control all those muscles you chose to relax and release them. Your body knows that relaxing the jaw...relaxes the hips...important knowledge as you prepare for this baby's birth. Releasing and relaxing the jaw with just a thought and a breath...breathing in relaxation and letting go of tension.

In this wonderfully relaxed state, give yourself permission to tune into your body and listen to your baby. Start your gentle conversations with this exciting new person as you begin your journey together.

You have the freedom and responsibility to nurture your body and that of your baby's. You are learning to trust that inner wisdom...gaining all the knowledge you can to create a safe and healthy environment for you and your child. Nurturing the body, plus the mind, with good foods and good positive thoughts about yourself, your partner and of course, baby. Communicating your love for them physically, verbally and with your heart. Preparing not only your body with the exercise it needs but also nurturing your mind with the knowledge that you do hold both that responsibility and freedom to take the best care possible of this body of yours. It is this body that provides the nutrients and oxygen to your child. This body needs and deserves your respect and care. Honour it for what it is..."the mother of your child".

Building a strong foundation...preparing that foundation physically, mentally and instinctively for the birth of your child. Bringing your awareness to these foundations... braiding them together, making the whole stronger than the pieces. Your baby needs all the pieces to the puzzle.

Take a deep, deep breath and gently blow out through your lips...releasing all negative thoughts, as you breathe in confidence and faith in your body and your inner wisdom. You relax deeply and completely with the knowledge that centuries of strong women's genes are guiding your body and baby in harmony. Listening to the powerful bond you have with this child allowing yourself to become more connected with each breath. Strengthen your posture to aid in this harmonious relationship...remember to plant your feet like a tree your weight dropping down into down into your heels creating that solid foundation for your growing baby. Like a tree...extend your spine... the roots to the earth, the upper body like branches to the sky, giving baby room to grow.

When you are sitting or lying down, use this same feeling in your pelvis, allow it to become heavy and grounded, letting your lower spine relax and your upper body elongate ...inviting in that all important grounding. Securing your foundation, permitting the rest of you to become lighter and freer. And as you become lighter, notice how aware you are of your baby. Notice how still your mind is as you focus your awareness inwards...connecting with your body and your baby. Work each breath like a natural wave...directing your exhalation downwards with gravity towards your "roots" while your inhalations lift lightly upwards toward your sun, lengthening your spine.

Allow this breath to become natural, feel the balance and serenity that it brings. Instinctively follow your body's rhythm with your breath become aware of your breathing. Trust your inner wisdom believe in your body and your baby. Aid your body with each breath... and visualize the oxygen flowing where it is needed, releasing any fears and anxieties that need letting go. Listening to your body, trusting it to do what is needed when the time for baby to join you on the outside is right...tuning in to your natural mommy instincts.

As you relax and release your body, your mind also relaxes and opens...allowing you to visualize or imagine whatever you choose.

Imagine or visualize yourself on a warm beach, a beach of your choosing, one with gentle waves softly moving up and back just beyond the spot you are laying. Listen to the waves and note their soft rhythm. Listen intensely to all the sounds around you; notice they do not disturb you in any way. Allow yourself to breath effortlessly and lightly....completely feeling everything in your body...communicating the calm, gentle feelings you share with your baby. Listen to the quiet between the waves...anticipate the movement of the water...looking for and finding the rhythm.

Listen to the waves; they are coming closer and closer, slowly coming in just beyond your feet. Feel the gentle touch of the water on your feet, notice you have no fear or concern...you are so safe and relaxed. There is no need to draw away from the water. The water is warm just the way you like it...smooth, comforting and calming.

 As the next wave moves over your feet you breathe in and as it recedes you breathe out...opening every part of your body, finding that perfect flow. Release all tension from your body as you exhale. And complete relaxation on the inhale. In harmony...your mind, body and baby working together... allowing nature to direct you both. The warm nurturing waves continue to comfort your body as they move over your body. With each wave you breathe and become more relaxed and open. Before long the waves have gently and safely carried you into the water...supporting you perfectly and completely.

You now relax in the warm, peaceful weightlessness of the ocean, that sea of your imagination. With each exhale you relax deeper and feel more supported and comforted by the water. As you are gently carried by the waves you breathe deeper, exhale completely, with each breathe and exhale you relax more deeply, your body opens further with each wave. The movement brings you comfort, the waves are pleasurable; you relax and breathe with each wave.

The wave intensifies...you breathe...and exhale.

The wave is powerful...you breathe...and exhale.

The wave strengthens...you breathe...and exhale.

The wave flows...you breathe...and exhale.

You control your breath and your rhythm. You find that perfect harmony with your body and your breath. The wave eventually comes back to the beach...you breathe...The wave is quiet...you breathe...exhaling completely...The wave is calm...you breathe...and exhale.

You see yourself lying on the warm soft sand. Peacefully and calmly breathing with the cycle, knowing it is a cycle of life...You and your infant are a part of that cycle...this brings you joy.

The wave recedes...you breathe...and exhale.

You feel the energy within you; you are completely in tune with your body and your baby. You have found harmony in your breathing and have made the mind-body connection....remaining beautifully calm and relaxed, trusting yourself, your intuition and the nature of the birthing process. You are able to rest more peacefully and comfortably for the exact amount of time required by your body for your baby, venting and releasing anything that needs to be during your dreamtime...knowing it is wise to in birth as in life to "expect normal but to accept the unexpected". You are listening carefully to your baby and your body and nature...wisely preparing for the best possible birth.

Chapter 3   Healing

Glowing Restoration

by Jeannie Rudyk

First of all, I would like you to find a place on the wall or the ceiling. A place to focus on. A place that is comfortable to you. It is comfortable but still challenging your eyes to focus upwards. Allow yourself to relax. Focusing on the spot.. challenging your eyes. Allowing yourself to relax. Allow your body to relax.

You're finding your body is relaxing now. I am going to count back from five to one. You are going to find yourself relaxing deeper and deeper. As we move from five to one finding yourself moving deeper down. Five...the weight of your eyes getting heavier...but still focusing on the spot. Four...finding your legs relaxing...and your arms are relaxing. Challenging your eyes to focus. Feeling your body relaxing now...Three...all the muscles around your face are loosening and unwinding. Two...you're still focused on the spot but your eyes are getting heavy and it is harder to keep them open. One...allowing your eyes to close completely. You are completely relaxed now. And anytime that you hear my voice saying *deeper* or *relaxed*, you find that it becomes easier to relax and go deeper.

You are completely relaxed...completely relaxed now...you are at the top of a beautiful set of stairs...and these stairs are exactly what you need to see at this moment in time...you can see a beautiful garden setting below...like a wonderful, mystical forest below...you feel drawn to this forest...moving towards the forest...you find your body relaxing... ten...finding your body becoming more relaxed...nine..you're body is becoming delightfully heavy...eight...all of the noises around you are fading away...all of the noises around this room are helping you relax deeper...deeper down...deeper relaxed...seven...anything you hear in this room or out of the room causes you to relax deeper...six...moving down, down, deeper and deeper into yourself...five...noticing your breathing has changed and you are more relaxed... four...your body feeling heavy. Delightfully heavy now... three...all the muscles in your body are relaxed...you may even feel a small tingling sensation in your hands...and feet...two...breathing deep...and every time you exhale you find yourself relaxing deeper. One...almost there now...and zero...finding yourself in the garden now...feeling the ground beneath your feet...

Feeling the healing energy of this garden...you can see the dew in the grass around you...and you can see the breeze swaying the trees back and forth...and as these trees sway back and forth....you can smell the trees and the grass and the air...breathing them in..and every time these trees sway back and forth you find yourself relaxing deeper and deeper down...noticing in the distance...there is another set of stairs...and you are drawn to these stairs...seeing another beautiful garden in the distance...down and down...you are relaxing...you can feel the wind is blowing...you can hear the breeze through the grass nearby...it is a warm comforting breeze. Walking along this beautiful path, running your hands along the tall grass as you go, every step relaxing more.

(Depending on the person, I may test for depth and do more deepening here.)

Finding yourself at these stairs, going down. And as you go down you find yourself relaxing deeper, deeper still. Twice as deep as before...five...going down...four...relaxing your body...three....finding yourself drawn to this place...two... feeling your breathing change, relaxing and slowing even more now, one and five...four...Allowing, letting go... three....relaxing...feeling your breathing...two and one...

Five...four...three...relaxing...two...allowing yourself to let go...and one....there now...there, in this garden you can feel your whole body letting go now...looking up into the sky, you can feel the sun against your face...so relaxing...so relaxing against your face...breathing in the clean, crisp air, the heat of the sun penetrating down against your face...so comforting, so warm, so healing. This light is any colour that you need for your healing now.

The sun is moving toward you now, coming down...down, deeper, your body is relaxing. And the sun moves towards your body, like a big, beautiful healing dome. Any colour that you need. Any colour that you need for your healing. You find yourself relaxing more and more, deeper, and deeper. Five...coming closer, four...feeling the radiance rain down, so relaxing, so comforting, three...down...two...closer still, and... one.

The sun is right in front of you now. The rays are washing over your body like waves. You are seeing all the colors on your body...feeling and seeing the colours move down your body. Feeling the heat, the light, on the crown of your head, moving down, over your forehead, over your eyes...relaxing all the tiny muscles in your eyes, and around your eyes. Down your cheeks, around your jaw...causing your mouth to open slightly, allowing your body to breathe. Down your neck and over your shoulders, releasing all the tension through the muscles in your back, all the muscles of your chest and over your stomach. The rays of the wonderful healing heat running over one arm...then the other. Rolling over your hips and exploding out like a giant ribbon...wrapping your body in healing energy. Around your hips and down one leg, then the other. Feeling the heat on the tops of your feet, flowing under your feet. This giant wave of heat wrapping around you, releasing any pain or hurt now. Breathing in the sun, breathing in the rays of colour. Deep, deep down into your body. Healing your body. Bring the colour into your body, taking it into every cell, into every cell of your entire being.

You are laying down...the rays of light, enveloping you. The sun moving closer to you still, taking you into its center. You can feel all the energy of the sun. If you feel any area on your body needing healing, the light is concentrating there now. Breathing in the sun, taking the sun into your body. Feeling your body filling with life and energy. All the pain washed away from your body. Energy revitalizing your body, sinking into your skin. Wrapped up in the energy cocoon.

You know now, that you can come to this energy anytime you want. It is in your body, you have taken it in. Every time you see the sun, you can feel it again. Every time you feel yourself losing this energy, you can reach within yourself...visualize the sun, taking in the sun every day. The colours of the sun wrapping around your body like a warm blanket. Feeling the sun deep within your being, you can let me know when you are ready to move forward.

The sun begins to drift, drift up into the air. Swaying in the warm breeze...carrying you to a wonderful little pond. Feeling the sun drifting down slowly, with a light sway...back and forth, back and forth, bringing you down. Five...down. Four...relaxing you further down. Three...moving, drifting. Two...down, down, deeper down, almost there now, and... one...placing you gently down on the beach. Taking a moment to look at this magical place around you. Taking in all the colours and the sounds. And taking a deep breath of the clean air. Smelling the grass and the flowers.

Looking down the beach, you notice a big, beautiful mirror... moving towards the mirror you can start to see all the little details of the mirror. Taking them in. Feeling the beach beneath your feet as you walk towards the mirror. Noticing the sun following behind you, the comforting warmth at your back. Looking into the mirror you can see yourself, like a movie playing though the magical glass. Any feelings your subconscious mind wants to work on now appear and you can see these things now.

Do you see them now?

Take a look at these things and how they were caused, knowing you are safe here...just watching from a distance, through the mirror...Safe here with the sun, just watching it, through the mirror. Feeling the warm sun at your back. Watch yourself in the mirror, your expression, as the scene plays out. When you are ready, reach through the mirror with just one arm, and feel the feelings of that time, just for a moment. You can take back your arm at any time.

When you are ready...just let me know.

You can do that now, in this moment, moving your hand

forward, connecting to the feelings there...these feelings you carry. This will help you understand the power of your subconscious mind. You will be able to pull your arm back at any time. You can feel that emotion, that time in the mirror... just for a moment...feeling your mind bringing these emotions back to you now...

Taking your hand back to your body, you can turn and place your hand into the sun, even stepping into that warm, beautiful sun. Allowing all those feelings to melt away. Knowing now, the power of your thoughts and emotions and how they feel in your body. Letting it all wash away in the rays of the sun again. Safe here...healed here. The ribbons of energy wrapping around you, healing all that was in the mirror. Those rays of the sun, exploding with healing energy around you. Letting go of those feelings now. Take a deep breath, breathing in the colors the sunlight, breathing and healing, breathing in that healing energy...deep, deep down into every cell, every fibre. Knowing now that you can intensify those feelings with thoughts and images in your mind, but you also have the power to feel relaxed, healed and energized. Just as you are in the sun. Now...breathing in the rays of the sun. Breathing in now. Exhaling any worries or pains, breathing in the healing.

Feeling safe to step back out of the sunlight now, you walk toward the mirror, looking down, you find a large rock...picking it up, you can feel the weight of all those feelings from that mirror, heavy...lifting it higher and higher, above your head. Throwing it at the mirror...the mirror shatters, it explodes...exploding into tiny pieces like dust. You can hear the explosion, feel it...all full of colors, crashing down...the frame that was holding the mirror comes down in pieces, all crashing down into dust. Small little pieces of dust and fragments. You can see the mirror and all those tiny colors, broken down...all those feelings in pieces. Feeling the sun at your back, there for you if you need it. You can step back into the sunlight if you need to...

You feel a warm breeze coming up from behind you. Whether you are in the sunlight or outside of it, you can feel the breeze. Feeling it toss your hair around. This wind is a warm, calming wind. It almost feels like a kind wind. This wind wraps around you, cradles you in its warmth, then whips away toward the shattered mirror, picking it up like a whirlwind...all the little pieces, all the little fragments, being carried up. Up into the air, further and further from you. You can feel it in your body, being carried away, from your body and from your mind. All those feelings drifting away. Feeling your body relax, as the fragments drift further away from you. Five...relaxing more and more...four...feeling all those feelings fade...three...all the energy of the sun within you. Two...the dust and fragments barely visible in the distance. One...like a speck in the sky, and zero...your whole body releasing those old feelings...they are gone in the wind. Carried far, far away from you. Your body turns into the sun, enveloping you. (*Start with compounding*)

Feeling yourself now inside the sun. Breathing in all the colours, all the healing energy. The delightful heat. Feeling rested and relaxed. Knowing now that you are inside of the sun, and as you breathe in the sun...it is inside of you. The sun is with you every day, and you can visualize the sun if you ever need to relax and feel this good again. Breathing in all its energy, and every time you breathe in, you can feel the energy inside you grow. Spreading throughout your body. Feeling so good. So relaxed, yet so full of energy. This energy you can bring into your everyday life. It is with you now, like the sun and the heat, and all the healing. Every time you think of the colours of the sun, in your mind, you feel this good. The energy coming from within you. (*Any more compounding*)

The sun starts to gently lift off, moving towards my voice. Moving towards this room. And in a moment I will count from one to ten and you will open your eyes, feeling relaxed and so alive with energy. One...all pains gone, two...feeling amazingly energized from head to toe, three...knowing the heat of the sun, and healing energy is within your body, and within your mind, four...feeling that healing energy, five... moving closer, six...knowing you can visualize that sunlight whenever you need, seven...starting to hear sound around you, becoming more aware, eight...feeling your body waking, feeling that energy within, nine...knowing you have that energy, that sunlight, 10...opening your eyes now...

Connecting to Your Source

By Angie J. Hernandez

As a hypnotherapist, I realized that as I strived to meet my clients where they were, I was constantly tripping over where they had been. I wanted a method to connect to those past moments when they felt unsupported, betrayed, or maybe even stunned by their own behavior. I didn't want to revisit their most traumatic moments but I did want to discharge the strong feelings that were left behind. I felt these highly emotionally charged events were stepping in the way of my clients' pursuit to better themselves and achieve new goals.

I developed this method I call "Connecting to Your Source" and it begins in your pre-talk:

"I don't see auras but I've been told by those who do, that there are energy cords connecting one person to another. These cords hook up whenever we encounter another person. I see them in my mind as big, fat electrical cords that are plugged in between me and you. I picture them as transparent cables with colored streams of energy.

Now, I know these energy cords exist because we've all had people that make us feel energized! We just feel great whenever we're around them. Then there are others that completely drain us of our energy. I know you know someone like that! Someone you avoid because talking to them leaves you feeling weak and out of sorts. It feels like they have sucked all the energy out of you!

The best encounter is when you exchange energy and you both come out feeling positive and happy. We also have energy cords that connect us to our Source. The Source, for some people, is God. For others, the Source may be called their Higher Power. Others still, may just think of the Source as their Intuition or Inner Voice. Whatever you call it, you have an energy cord that connects you to your Source. When you need support, the Source sends to energy to help you get through. But there have been times in everyone's life when they felt that connection was broken or damaged. These times might have left you feeling disconnected or alone, your energy cord in bad shape or even broken.

So what we want to do today is repair those cords between you and your Source, during those times of trauma, to discharge the strong emotions surrounding those times. When you've healed the cords, you will find yourself feeling freer and easier in your mind and body. This allows you to move forward making the changes you told me you want to achieve."

At this point you may begin your hypnosis as you choose. When your client is in trance and you see them very relaxed, you may begin in this way.

Imagine yourself, as you are right now; yourself in the present moment. And notice reaching out in one direction, away from you, is a ribbon that represents your past. You can see it stretching out from you and you notice that there are happy times and some traumatic times. But we're not going to experience those feelings now. Just note that they are there and that they do not cause you to react in any way. They are just there and you are very relaxed.

Also note that in the other direction, stretches another ribbon that represents your future. It is a golden ribbon that stands for your future prosperity and well being. You can notice that it stretches well into the future.

But as you come back to the present moment, you can look above your head and you'll see an energy field flowing above you. Now, this isn't the kind of energy that when you touch it, you feel an electric shock. This is the kind of energy that fills you up and re-energizes you. It feels wonderful; so soothing and inspiring at the same moment. Go ahead, reach your hands up and touch it. Doesn't it feel wonderful? I don't even know how to describe it myself, but you know...tell me how that feels to you... (*pause until your client speaks an answer, repeat what they say and remark upon it.*)

That is part of the energy from your Source. It's there to nourish you, to fill you and sustain you. It refreshes you and gives you what you need in tough circumstances. I don't know what is the most important to you, whether it's the strength you get from it or the nourishment of your soul and body or maybe just the wonderful connected way you feel.

And now let's move out over your timeline, into the past. I just want you to float over your timeline. You won't experience any past events, but you'll see where they are. Way down on the ribbon of the timeline, are all those events of your past and you see them as you float back in time. Float back over the days, over the months and over the years. I want you to float way back to the time you were conceived in your mother's womb.

Now, I will say your age to you. I want you to look at the timeline and raise your finger if you notice any events where

85

the energy cord between you and your Source is either broken or damaged. Here we go:

From conception to birth: *(wait to see if the finger lifts in an Ideomotor Response)*

Birth to age 5: *(again wait, if there is a response to either time, note that as we will come back to it)*

If there has been any response to these two time periods, proceed like this:

OK, let's go back.

First trimester

Second trimester

Third trimester

Age 1

Age 2

Age 3

Note the ages where your client gives the IR of raising their finger. Then proceed.

Let's go to the age of two. Look down at your timeline and reach to the energy cord from this age. Do you have it? Good. Now look at the cord for where it is damaged. You can see that the energy from your Source cannot move smoothly through this damaged cord. Maybe it's broken and no energy at all can be given to your two year old self. Now reach up into the energy field above you and grab the part of the energy cord that's connected to your Source. Repair the two pieces of the cord. Reconnect them. Now smooth out the connection so it is smooth and functioning. You may need to stretch it straight and uncoil any kinks. When you have finished repairing the cord, make sure it is securely plugged into your two year old self. You still are not feeling any trauma or bad feelings from that time. That time is neutral to you. You're simply repairing the energy cord and allowing the energy from your Source to flow freely again.

Just give me a head nod when you've finished repairing the cord.

Now that the cord is repaired and energy flows freely from your Source, allow that energy to flow into your body. You can feel it nourishing and replenishing that which was lost. It fills you up and you can feel the peace flow into every cell. It energizes all the physical body's organs with a sense of well being that's been missing. You feel a new purpose and direction. That purpose sizzles within you.

When your body and mind are completely filled and nourished, raise your finger to let me know.

Wait for the finger to raise, it may take some time but be patient and allow however much time your client needs. Proceed to the next age your client indicated as damaged or broken. Repair that cord, as well. When there are no more cords to repair in the age sequence, proceed to the next set.

Age 4

Age 5

Age 6

Age 7

Age 8

Age 9

Age 10 (Note each age where an IMR occurred. Now go back to those ages and repair the cord.)

Reach down for the cord in your past and reach up for the cord from your Source. Lock them together and begin repairing the damage. That's right, smooth out the broken spots. Mold together the breaks. Smooth out and stretch the cord into a smooth connection. Let me know when the cord is like new and the energy from the Source is flowing smoothly...good, now feel the healing energy flowing into your body. You are thirsty for it. It nourishes you and fills you. You can feel it rushing to all those cells in your body that have needed it for so long. Allow it to reach every single cell of you, even your brain; it now begins to feed and complete in you what has been missing. And when you are filled completely and you feel well satisfied, let me know.

Continue through each year of your client's life. I ask for a response as we go through 5-10 years of age. Then I return to any year they indicated had a break or some damage to their energy cord. I give them time to repair the cord and time for the energy to re-fill the body and replenish what was lost. We do not experience any emotion from that time, we merely make note of it and then repair the cord, feeling the relief and healing that brings. I say it slightly different each time. Usually by the time we have repaired the cord several times, the process is quicker.

Now, we have repaired all the problems with your energy cords from the time you were conceived, until today. Look back over your timeline into the past and see all the work you have done. You can say to yourself, "I like that."

I don't know whether you will feel this in the next few hours or over the next couple of days, but you will notice that those memories that used to cause you such pain and anxiety, no longer feel so sharp. They will not have the sting they had in the past, in fact, you'll find you can think of those times and wonder why they bothered you so much before. That they could cause you any strong emotion will seem silly and you may find yourself grinning at how they used to make you feel. See, there's that little grin now.

In the next few days, you will find yourself venting out those old emotions and negative thoughts in vivid venting dreams. And you'll know your mind is cleaning house and releasing you from those old, outdated trains of thought. You'll feel a freedom and lightness that seems new to you but so welcome. I don't know if you're the kind of person that will value more the happy thoughts that come to you now so easily or the lightness in your step but this new way of thinking and that beautiful energy flow in you will make you see colors and light in a whole new way. You are stepping into the part of your life where happiness seems so easy for you.

Now, you may bring your client out in your usual way. They will feel lighter and less burdened by bad memories. My clients report that they still have the bad memories but the strong, emotional charge is gone. They can recall those times but without the sting.

Deep Peat 4 with Reiki

by Michele Cempaka

This innovative treatment, which was created by myself, combines the power of Reiki with energy psychology to assist people in clearing away phobias, past traumas or painful experiences that are affecting a person's life.

PEAT (Primordial Energy Activation & Transcendence) originates from a system of healing by Sivorard, a Serbian man who has done some amazing work with transforming individuals' consciousness and lives.

The practitioner begins by asking the client how much this issue bothers them from 0 - 10 with 10 being extremely challenging. She then guides the client to create a picture in their mind related to the issue that they would like to release, while the practitioner channels Reiki to the specific Chakras which correspond to this experience.

Four questions are posed to the client during the session to facilitate access to the person's subconscious as follows:

1. What do you see?
2. What are you thinking?
3. What are you feeling?
4. Do you have any sensations in your body right now?

The client answers two or more of these questions while touching the left inner eye with her two fingers; this stimulates both the kidney meridian and the subconscious where the memory of the event or fear is stored.

Next, the practitioner instructs the client to switch her fingers to the right inner eye and at this time the client either imagines a peaceful sanctuary, or for those who are more

pragmatic, they can just come back to the 'here and now'.
The practitioner then asks the same questions: What do you see? What are you thinking? What are you feeling? Do you have any sensations in your body right now?

The client responds and the process continues, with the client switching from their left to right eyes, with the practitioner repeating the same questions and channeling Reiki to the corresponding chakras...until the picture or feelings, thoughts and sensations totally disappear.

The practitioner checks again to be sure the issue has been cleared by asking the client from 0 - 10 how they would rate their issue? The optimum number is either 0 or 1. If anything higher than this, return to the protocol and continue until the issue has been totally cleared. The end result is total neutralization of the issue which is energetically released, restoring one's natural even-flow.

I have had a great deal of success with this system for clients with fears, phobias and even helped one client resolve PTSD. It has also been very successful for releasing deep anger and other emotional upsets.

The Pool by the Waterfall

By Birgit Wujcik

Anchoring stone/crystal/object to trigger confidence, control and calmness for anxiety and stress but easily adaptable for other issues.

Allow your client to choose a small crystal at the beginning of this session or bring in a stone or object (*jewelry*) of their choice. Encourage client to look at the stone/crystal/object, feel how it feels in their hand and then place it aside. Suggest to client that this stone/crystal/object can be worn on a necklace, hung on a car mirror or key chain.

Begin with an appropriate induction, deepener and suggest a nature scene. Guide your client to a cleansing waterfall and describe the large pool at the foot of the waterfall. Allow client to cleanse under the waterfall and walk, swim or float to the other end of the large pool where he may sit on a rock or bench or grass...or take your client on a nature walk through the forest where he finds a large pond or lake.

You can barely see the waterfall in the distance and faintly hear the sound of the water as it feeds into the large pool. Breathe in the fresh air as you walk close to the edge and gaze upon the water. The surface of the water is very still; sometimes there are ripples or even waves carried over by the wind from the waterfall...but for now the surface is very still, almost as still as a mirror. This pool represents your mind...your conscious mind and your subconscious mind. Notice how easy it is to observe the surface of the water...as easy as it is to observe the thoughts of your conscious mind.

92

As you stand by the edge of the water you know that the environment and weather around the pool, such as a storm, change the appearance of the pool...A storm creates ripples and waves on the surface of the water...the rays of the sun warm the surface of the water and toxic spills such as oil poisons the water...but deep underneath the surface there is a perfect calmness...

Your mind is much the same...calm and happy thoughts warm your mind like the sunshine...angry and negative thoughts create disturbance to the balance within your mind...and self-destructive thoughts poison your mind. A stressful environment can create negative thoughts...(*insert client's negative thoughts and language patterns*) and promote unwanted feelings such as (*insert client's symptoms*).

Deep within your subconscious mind there is peace, calmness and positivity. Just like the pool by the waterfall...the deeper the water, the calmer it is. Activity on the outside does not affect the calmness at the bottom of the pool. Any stressors from the environment stay on the surface...Every level of the water flows into another...as does your mind communicate with all parts of who you are...

A constant flow of information...traveling through all layers of your mind to your body like the water in the pool mixing all levels...A storm might create disturbance and allow the poisons on the surface to enter deeper levels...just like some events in your life affect you more than others and occupy your mind longer...but notice that the bottom of the pool stays the same...No matter how strong the storm or how much oil is spilled...This is the same for your mind. Those deep levels of your subconscious mind stay calm, peaceful, positive, content and secure...When you are relaxed your subconscious mind communicates those calm, peaceful, positive messages to your body and you are able to let go of all negative feelings, thoughts, anxiety and stress.

At the beginning of our session I gave you a *(object)*. I want you to imagine yourself standing by the edge of that pool...feeling safe, secure, calm and at peace...holding onto this *(object)* ...Feel its weight and cool texture...and I wonder if you can recall the details of how this *(object)* looks...but it doesn't really matter...as all you have to do is just imagine it.

This *(object)* represents calmness, confidence and control ...As you are gazing into the crystal clear water of the pool...you drop your *(object)* into the water...hear the sound of the water...Notice the little ripples as they dance across the surface of the pool and imagine the little splash of water as your *(object)* begins to sink.

In your mind's eye, follow and watch your *(object)* as it drops deeper and deeper...down and down...until it safely comes to rest at the bottom of the pool. Imagine a soft glow radiating from your *(object)*...illuminating the water around it with a mysterious shimmer and sparkle.

As your *(object)* rests on the bottom of the pool it becomes a permanent part of your life...As it rests on the bottom of the pool it communicates calmness, confidence and control to your body...especially during stressful situations.

Every time you see or hold your *(object)*...it triggers feelings of calmness, confidence and control...and all anxiety and stress *and* all symptoms of anxiety and stress will be replaced with a profound feeling of relaxation.

Mending Broken Heartstrings:
A Healing for Abortion or Miscarriage

by Shannon King

*(Use induction and deepeners of your choice, and take client to a peaceful place of their design. The words in normal font are read for healing from an abortion, and words that are **bold** are for healing from a **miscarriage**.)*

So now, just allow your conscious awareness to rest in this peaceful place, this place of your own design. This is a place that brings you comfort, a place that brings you relaxation, and a place where you can find healing. And you've come here today and you can find healing and forgiveness because you've come here to find healing and forgiveness.

(This section is specific for healing from abortion)

And as your conscious awareness finds rest and relaxation, your subconscious is right here to help you find the healing you are seeking. At some time in the past, you made a decision...because at the time this decision felt like the best decision for you. Because of the situation, or timing, or any other reason, you made a decision to terminate a pregnancy. And this may have been the best decision for you to make. Knowing you make decisions with the best of intention...now is a time to allow yourself to look at the positive intention for your decision.

Take a moment and ask your subconscious to gently show you what your positive intention was at that time...and as you just allow the feelings, thoughts, and emotions that accompany that decision and the positive intention behind the decision...as you just allow the feelings to come up...allow yourself to feel those feelings. These feelings are ok, and you're safe just allowing those feelings to be here for a moment. And just allow any thoughts that come into your awareness to just be...let them just float through you mind without judgment, just be aware the thought is there and let it float. And if there are any emotions that you are experiencing, just allow the emotions to be there...

Allow yourself to embrace the knowledge that at the time you made your decision you made it with positive intention...and any feelings, thoughts, or emotions that are no longer beneficial to you that no longer serve any purpose...acknowledge that they were there as a result of your decision and you can now let them go. If there is a feeling or indication of a need for forgiveness...a forgiveness of yourself or asking for forgiveness...then allow that to happen now.

Allow yourself to let those feelings, thoughts, and emotions to gently float away, floating up...floating away...until they are growing smaller and smaller...lighter and lighter...dimmer and dimmer...until they completely disappear...completely gone...no longer needed. And as you feel the peace and release from the burden of these old feelings, thoughts, and emotions, allow yourself to experience the beginning of acceptance and healing ...acceptance and healing, with the knowledge that you made your decision with positive intention at that time.

And because you have released those feelings that are no longer needed or beneficial to you, and found any forgiveness you might have needed...you are now experiencing healing and acceptance, a healing that is beneficial and needed...you will find that the feelings and emotions of healing and acceptance will continue to grow and develop because these are now your positive intentions.

(*This section in bold is specific for healing from a miscarriage*)

And as your conscious awareness finds rest and relaxation, your subconscious is right here to help you find the healing you are seeking. At some time in the past, you have experience the loss of you child during a pregnancy. And sometimes we know the reason of the miscarriage...and sometimes we do not...and it is difficult for us to understand why the miscarriage happened because the loss is the same. And it really does not matter the reason because the loss is the same. Although we cannot change the past...you can find healing in the present.

And that is what you are here to do right now...to find healing and acceptance. You cannot change the past...and you can find healing and acceptance in the present. Take a moment and ask your subconscious to gently show you any feelings and emotions you might have due to this loss...and as you just allow the feelings, thoughts, and emotions that accompany the loss of your child you might discover feelings and emotions that you were not aware of before...as you just allow the feelings to come up...allow yourself to feel those feelings.

These feelings are ok, and you're safe just allowing those feelings to be there for a moment. And just

allow any thoughts that come into your awareness to just be...let them just float through you mind without judgment, just be aware the thought is there and let it float. And if there are any emotions that your are experiencing, just allow the emotions to be there...

Allow yourself to embrace the knowledge that these feelings, these emotions and thoughts are OK...and some of these may no longer be beneficial for you. Some of these feelings, emotions, and thoughts, which began as a response to your loss and hurt and having no understanding of why your miscarriage happened, may no longer serve you and your higher purpose. And any feelings, thoughts, or emotions that are no longer beneficial to you, that no longer serve any purpose...acknowledge that they were there as a result of your loss and you can now let them go. Allow yourself to let those feelings, thoughts, and emotions that are no longer beneficial to gently float away, floating up...floating away...until they are growing smaller and smaller...lighter and lighter...until they completely disappear...they are completely gone...no longer needed.

And as you feel the peace and release from the burden of these old feelings, thoughts, and emotions, allow yourself to experience the beginnings of acceptance and healing...acceptance and healing, with the knowledge that the past is in the past, and the present is here.

And because you have released those feelings that

are no longer needed or beneficial to you, and you are now experiencing healing and acceptance, a healing that is beneficial and needed, you will find that the feelings and emotions of healing and acceptance will continue to grow and develop because these are now what you need.

And as you allow these feelings of healing and acceptance to just flow through you, entirely through your body, and mind, and soul,...if you choose you can ask your inner wisdom, or higher power, or God to show to you the child that you let go (**lost**). If you choose this at this time, indicate by raising an index finger.

(If the indication is yes) ~ Good. Go ahead and ask your inner wisdom, or higher power, or God to show to you the child that you let go (**lost**). And as this child comes to you, you may say anything to this child that you want to say...and you may hold or hug this child if you choose...and you might ask or give this child a name. Take a few moments to just be with this child and find any answers you might need...tell this child anything you want...and just connect with this child in a way that is healing to you...Allow yourself to embrace this child from your new position of acceptance and healing. And when you are done, just let me know by nodding your head.

(Pause and allow the client time to process.) Wonderful...now as you are still with this child, see or feel the heartstring that once connected both of you...a beautiful heartstring of any color. See or feel this heartstring coming from your heart and allow this heartstring to re-connect with your child's beautiful heartstring. Feel the healing and peace as this heartstring mends...connecting your hearts together

again. Knowing that you are OK...knowing that your child is OK...knowing that your heartstring is mended and you can remember or connect on a spiritual level with this child whenever you chose. The past is gone and now is the time for healing and acceptance. Now is the time to just let your heart and soul to embrace this connection and healing for both you and your child.

Take a nice deep breath and as you exhale...just feel the feelings of peace that comes with this healing...feel the joy that comes from your new acceptance...feel the love that comes with the mending of the heartstring between you and your child. Just feel it. And now just allow yourself to take the time you need to complete this healing and finish anything else you need with this child. And when you are done, let me know by nodding your head.

(Awaken with positive post hypnotic suggestions and awakening of your choice.)

(If the indication is No) ~ Good. If you have found the healing and forgiveness that you have come here to find and are contented and at peace, indicate a positive response by lifting an index finger.

(If the indication is yes, provide the client with positive post hypnotic suggestions and bring to alertness. If the indication is negative, ask the client if more healing is needed at this time or what she might need to accomplish that healing and proceed as appropriate.)

Forgiveness Script

by Andrea Hedley

This Forgiveness Script is for clients who are suffering from resentment arising from real or perceived wrongdoings by others. A person may feel angry or hurt in the moment, but if they are revisiting that hurt over and over in their mind, it becomes resentment. They are re-experiencing that pain on a consistent basis, often leading to depression, anxiety, or the very real health impacts of carrying persistent hostility. When we forgive, we free ourselves from reliving past events. We allow ourselves to live in the present moment instead of in the past, leading to healing and often empathy for ourselves and others.

I'd like you to imagine that you are standing in a dark room except for one area in the centre of the room that is illuminated. Imagine that the person who has hurt you is standing in the illuminated area. As you observe them standing there, bring to mind what they did to you. Think of all of the qualities that you resent, that make you angry, everything they've done that has made life difficult for you.

Now visualize that this energy is radiating out of the person in a red negative light. Imagine this red light coming towards you, a red hurtful energy intended to harm. You might even be able to feel its heat as it hits you.

Imagine that you, in turn, are triggered by this energy and it creates a red hurtful band of energy inside of you, radiating back to the other person. Then watch it return to you again and see the red negative band of energy going back and forth, back and forth as the pain-trigger-response cycle continues. Maybe you can understand that if one of you doesn't choose to stop returning the energy that this pattern will continue on endlessly.

Now decide that you are going to stop sending the red energy back to them. Let all of that person's hurt, resentment, anger radiate towards you, feeling the full force of their ill will. Take some time to let yourself experience how they have hurt you and what does pain their actions have caused.

Now imagine that a white healing light originates within you as a result of your decision not to participate in returning negative energy. See a white light coming from within you and flowing through you and around you. Then bring your attention back to that red energy flowing towards you, but this time visualize that when the hurtful band of red energy meets the white, it just runs off of you in rivulets, dissolving. It can no longer trigger you. See that red energy just running down into the ground. The white light is refreshing you as it clears out the remnants of the pain inside of you, leaving you feeling open and peaceful. Take a deep breath and enjoy your decision not to engage in the cycle of pain. Now imagine this white light and the commitment to peace that it represents is surrounding you, radiating out for a few feet around your entire body. This refreshing white light is protecting you and the band of red energy cannot penetrate it. In the future if you see this person, you will imagine this white light surrounding you, dissolving any negativity that is directed at you.

Again, focus your attention on this person and that hurtful red energy they hold within them. Then take a moment to see if there is anything going on underneath that hurtful red energy...if there are other issues such as pain or loss that may be creating some of their negative emotions. As you look at this person in their pain or anger, perhaps stuck in their issues, imagine that the white light floods toward and through them. Imagine that this white light is an act of forgiveness healing them, healing their grievances and their pain. The whole room is flooded in this light, purifying and clarifying.

Next, visualize someone that represents the principals of forgiveness to you there in the room with you. This could be a religious or political figure or someone in your own life who lives by the principles of forgiveness (Buddha, Nelson Mandela, Jesus). Observe them, observe their energy, and see how they embody those principles. Try to imagine what their response would be to the person that hurt you.

Now imagine that others who are committed to forgiveness - from throughout history or from the present day - are joining this figure, they are joining hands and surrounding you and the other person, encircling you. Take a moment to see how this forgiveness is for you. That it exists and grows within you regardless of the other person's actions or path to healing. You may wish for them to find a path of healing their pain or confusion, but you recognize that you have no control over their choices.

All of these individuals are surrounding you and supporting you in your decision to chose forgiveness, reminding you to return to the path of forgiveness each and every day, even when it's difficult, even when you are challenged, or hurt. They remind you that you are strong enough to feel the pain and still, return to forgiveness.

Now I'd you to imagine that you step back into the inner most circle, joining hands and becoming a part of it. Enjoy this feeling. Enjoy a sense of resolution, a commitment to forgiveness flowing through your hands. You look at the person of focus in the centre of the circle. You silently send them your empathy and compassion, and wish them healing, hoping that they will join the circle someday.

Magical Moon Experience

by Kelley T. Woods

I designed this mindful hypnosis script to help you find relief from any negative feelings, sensations or energies that the lunar cycle may be triggering in you. Use it to begin to change the way the mind and body react to the full moon...to instead imprint upon the unconscious mind...the positive connections and influences of our Mother Moon...which is an inspiration for our intuition and our creative imagination.

As you begin to settle yourself there...you might want to begin with taking a nice, deep and slow breath...and then, letting it out easily...knowing that just breathing in this way...slow...and easy...is a cue...a cue for your body to begin to release tension...a cue for your mind to begin to turn inward...that's right...just breathing effortlessly...and it is easy, isn't it...to begin to let go in this manner...because breathing is the one thing which we do from the moment we arrive in this world...to the last breath we take...so you could begin to imagine that as you inhale, you feel a wonderful wave of comfort move into and through your body and your mind...and as you exhale...any remaining tension dissipates...in fact, you could even begin to imagine that you are floating...gently floating somewhere...feeling supported...safe...almost as if you are lying on a perfect cloud bed...up there...it's easy to float and even drift...if you want...drift even higher...to a vantage point where, up there, you can begin to see things from a different perspective... because it's impossible to see how things look down there until you allow yourself to float...above...and look down...

And perhaps it will help if you illuminate the scene...bring a gentle, glow to it...like that of the light of the moon... moonlight is a special light, isn't it? Especially the light of the full moon, in the light of the full moon, drifting up there, safe...you can take a look at things now and fully see them, clearly...

And then you can even begin to turn your thoughts about the thoughts and the feelings that are related to a full moon....for instance, you may not have known that the moon represents our deepest personal needs, our unconscious minds and our instinctive, emotional reactions...When we are positively inspired by the Moon, we are creative, intuitive, sentimental, adaptable, introspective, and protective. If negatively inspired, we become moody, restless and irrational...

The things we just seem to *know* without giving them any thought, such as our instincts, intuitive impulses, and hunches are all products of the Moon...

The forms of expression that you feel seem to emanate from your deepest self belong to the Moon, which can include all forms of art, letters, and creative work of any kind. By showing us our unconscious responses, the Moon helps us to gain deep personal insight and we can then work toward healing any deep emotional wounds we have experienced. By healing these wounds, we can then be free to grow into our authentic, powerful selves.

She is magic, she is mystery, and she is grace...she is both our inner child and our outer Mother...

And of course, there are many stories and fables and song and even poems about the moon...like that one called Goodnight Moon...by Margaret Wise Brown, who must be a very wise woman...

(Read Goodnight Moon here – you can easily find it online if you don't have this classic....)

And I wonder, when you think of that little book, which helps so many little children fall sweetly asleep, if you can imagine saying goodnight to all of your troubles, too...just letting them drift away as you drift deeper into this experience...perhaps also falling into a dream where you hear a lovely song that talks about amore...and you notice that part in it, where that deep and beautiful Italian voice sings...when the moon hits your eye, like a big piece o' pie...that's amore...and the thought of that fills your heart...your loving and happy heart fills with joy and wonder...at the thought of all of that moon-lit amore...and when you breathe it in...it feels even more wonderful...

I don't know if that's actually an Italian singing that song about amore...sometimes I suspect it might be the Man in the Moon and I remember a cloudless night when I was young and out for a walk with a lover...and we both looked up in unison at the full moon and for the first time ever, it seemed, I saw the Man in the Moon. He was smiling and looked so peaceful that I felt a wave of serenity come over me...so that it felt like I was walking on air...that night...under the light of the moon...with the man in the moon watching over me...

But time passed like it does and here we are now...with you relaxing there on your bed of cloud...smiling now with the thought of a happy heart and a peaceful mind...but what if I told you about the mouse that ran up the clock...hickory, dickory dock...and we know how fun that nursery rhyme is...with a dish running away with a spoon...and a little boy laughing...but my favorite part is when the cow jumps over the moon...what a sight that is...what spirit that cow has...to be able to jump over the moon...a playful spirit...that comes to mind whenever you think of the full moon...and the cow jumping over it...

Because now, you see...and understand, that the moon and especially the full moon is filled with many marvelous things for you...like a happy heart and a peaceful mind and a playful spirit...and when you say goodnight to any negative things, all of these gifts are just waiting for you...you may even like to embrace your own feminine aspect, whenever that beautiful moon is nearing...

Allow her to express herself fully in the most positive ways, through the inspiration of poetry, the emotion you feel while gazing into the eyes of a lover, and those mystifying instincts that can gently beckon you to places as yet unexplored. The mystical and magical depths is where you'll find her, how will you answer her irresistible call? The choice, as always, is yours.

As you drift there...let yourself rise up even higher...into the glorious light of that full moon...allow that light to permeate gently, softly, soothingly...healing any discord, removing any dis-ease...filling you throughout with a peaceful, yet invigorating sense of well being...and each breath that you take reminds you of these wonderful sensations, so that whenever you want or need, you can instantly bring them back, by breathing in this way and thinking of the beautiful moon, with all of her lovely aspects...

The Healing Shirt

by Monique Wilson

Use this comforting process to help clients who experience chronic pain and/or chronic stress. I take my time with this one...long pauses...and allow deep relaxation and the sensation of warmth to guide them to that healing place within.

Inhaling peace and relaxation, you then exhale tension...Releasing stress and going deeper into relaxation with each breath.

Your body is completely relaxed and in this relaxed state you reach for a shirt... imagining a soft, fleecy shirt. The shirt is light, and sooo soft. It is warm, in fact...it is so warm that it feels like a heating blanket...a heating blanket set at the perfect temperature for you, on this day.

Taking a nice deep breath, you slowly put your arm into the first sleeve; the soft fabric is soothing on your skin, and the heat causes your muscles to relax immediately. Your breath comes easier now, and the heat from the shirt wraps around your muscles, penetrating deep into your bones.

You feel all tension, all discomfort...lift out of your body. And you realize...that the shirt is absorbing all tension, all discomfort, all inflammation from your body. That this soft, comfortable, heated shirt is actually a healing shirt...

You take a nice deep breath and as you exhale, you release all discomfort into the shirt. And you continue to breathe deeply, so grateful to have such a soft warm sensation on your skin. The shirt collar is now resting on your neck, and the sleeve is wrapped around your shoulder. The heat is lifting, lifting, lifting...all inflammation...is being lifted out of your body and into the shirt.

You gently pull the shirt around your back, and as you do so...it softly clings to your skin and clothing...the heat is now relaxing all the muscles in your back, your shoulder blades, soothing as it gently molds to your body. The heat is perfect for this day...and you can feel the inflammation in your bones and muscles being lifted right up...out...and absorbed into the shirt.

Now you slowly slide your other arm into the sleeve, feeling the comforting heat...and breathing that deep relaxing breath, all tension being released.

You feel the heat soothing all of your back muscles, the vertebrae in your back releasing, becoming more flexible, more pliable...gently expanding their ability to move...Gently and slowly, you become more limber as the heat from the healing shirt soothes and lifts inflammation.

The shirt zips, buttons, or snaps...and it closes around your torso. You feel the heat penetrate your belly, soothing the organs...relaxing your digestive system...allowing it to reach the perfect state of balance. The heat soothes your lungs and heart, allowing you to breathe deeper, relax even deeper. Your liver, kidneys, your bowels...all release tension and stress...and as they release stress, they come into balance...functioning perfectly. The heat is sooo relaxing ...soothing...lifting all discomfort, all inflammation out of your body.

Slowly and gently you feel the heat begin to flow into your

pelvis and hips. Each joint is surrounded by the healing heat of the shirt...it clings to your lower back. All discomfort is absorbed by the shirt, and the soft heat gently heals and relaxes all the muscles in your lower back and buttocks. Breathing so easily now....

Your hips and joints become flexible and limber as the inflammation is lifted. As the heat flows into your legs you realize that the shirt is now becoming a suit...that this beautiful healing tool is expanding to your legs...wrapping around the muscles in your thighs, relaxing and releasing.

Your breath is deeply peaceful, and releases even more tension as the warmth flows into your knees...gently soothing and healing along the way. And finally, as your entire torso is filled with warmth and all inflammation is being gently pulled out of your body...your calves relax and release, letting of all that tension. Your body is completely relaxed now....

You notice, there in front of you, two gloves, two slippers and a hat. Each one is filled with soothing heat, of just the perfect temperature for you, on this day.

You slowly pull on one glove and as your fingers enter the glove, you feel the heat come in contact with your joints. Sweet comfort arrives and all inflammation is lifted...the perfect amount of healing for your body, on this day. The next hand is equally comforted by the calming heat...your hands are wrapped in soothing warmth.

And you gently slide on the slippers, and as you do you feel the heated slippers lift all discomfort and tension from your feet. Your joints are so calm now...and finally, you put on your hat. This time, the healing warmth of the hat lifts all remaining tension; any thoughts that represent stress...are lifted. The only awareness that you have is an awareness of balance and healing.

You gladly spend some time here now...Your entire body is wrapped in this healing suit. All tension is released, all stress is released. All inflammation is lifted out of your body. And for the next several minutes you ALLOW all inflammation to be lifted out and away from your body. This is the perfect amount of healing for you, at this time. And with each breath you feel calmer, more relaxed...you feel comfort and peace...Deeper, and deeper now....

At this point I add positive suggestions that reflect the goals that my client has expressed..."As you heal, you feel a strength growing from deep within you, generating energy, positive...healing energy."

Or..."As your body heals you see it gracefully moving, flowing with flexibility and strength. You now have the stamina to embark on the activities that you desire"...

Or, "As your body heals, your mind begins to clear and you see those creative ideas begin to blossom..."

A Journey through the Crystals

by Joy O'Dwyer

You can modify this script by experiencing the amethyst crystal and then just one other crystal, or two others, depending on the needs of your client and your time frame.

Take a deep breath...You are so relaxed now...Feel the relaxation throughout your whole body from the top of your head to the tips of your toes...You feel so safe and so relaxed...

Now imagine you are going on a journey of discovery. You open your left hand and see a beautiful amethyst crystal. It is oblong in shape, with one end larger than the other. It has rings of mauve, purple and white and is smooth to your touch. You feel the crystal getting warm in your palm. It is such a soothing sensation. You sense a pulsing energy at your base chakra at the tip of your spine. A spiralling energy moves slowly up your chakras, spinning to the top of your head. Feel the pulsing energy. It is relaxing and yet energizing. Enjoy the energy of the crystal as it invites you on a journey. (*Pause*)

The spiralling begins to calm you as your mind becomes more open and receptive. You see a flash of brilliant white light as you open to the crystal. Then you are standing on a pure white sand beach.

You feel the soft sand beneath your toes. The sun shines on you, warm and soothing. The beach seems familiar, like you have seen it in a dream somewhere beyond time. You look

113

across the broad expanse of water and see the sun rippling across the waves that gently touch the shoreline. You feel an incredible peace. You smile as the rays of the sun warm your mind and spirit.

You see someone in the distance walking towards you surrounded by white light. As this person comes closer you recognize this being as your spirit guide or guardian angel. She smiles at you with a radiance that permeates your whole body with peace. You understand that all is well as she whispers peace to your soul.

Your spirit guide disappears from view, and your gaze is drawn to your left. You see a twenty foot tall amethyst crystal sitting upright in the sand. The white and purple hues dazzle you with their beauty and symmetry. You look upward as you realize the height of the massive crystal. You are amazed at its size and beauty. The base is twice as large as the top and you realize that it is in the same shape as the crystal that you have in your palm.

You sit in a lotus position before the crystal. The dazzling colours of the amethyst shine upon you and permeate your body with a soft glow. You feel the healing power of the crystal. Breathe in the healing power of the crystal. (*Pause*)

A white light from above shines down over the crystal and encases you in its glow. You feel the healing power as it gently moves down through your body. You hear a soft voice speak to your mind. You know that it is from God. You listen intently to receive the message: "I created everything, including the crystals. They are part of my creations, which are endless. Be at peace."

You feel the healing energy of the white light and the crystal.

The message to be at peace reverberates throughout your mind and body. Be at peace. Be at peace. Be at peace. You breathe deeply into the essence of the amethyst knowing that you are healing body, mind and spirit. You gently bask in the presence of the crystal. You are beyond time and space and all is well. (*Pause*)

You take the crystal from your hand and place it at the base of the large crystal. You thank the crystal for its wisdom and insight. (*Pause*)

You continue your walk along the white sand beach, feeling peaceful and energized.

You notice a brilliant yellow light shimmering in the distance. You are curious to know what this could be and walk steadily toward it, mesmerized by the dazzling glow. As you get closer, you realize that the sand has become like tiny yellow crystals. You sink into the glistening yellow sand. As you quietly sit and breathe in the beauty of the surroundings, to your left you see a spinning crystal the same colour as the sand. It is angular, with several points. It reminds you of a triple pyramid as it spins slowly in front of you. You feel a healing energy from the crystal and bask in its presence. A voice in your mind tells you to put the crystal in the middle of your forehead. You take the crystal, lie down in the sparkling sand, and place it in the middle of your forehead. Another similar one suddenly appears, spinning before you. You place this one on your navel. A third appears and you know to place it on the area of your body which is in need of healing.

You breathe deeply. As you do, you feel the healing power of the crystals. You feel peaceful as you lie still on the sand, enjoying the radiating energy of the crystals. (*Pause*)

You hear a voice in your mind's eye which tells you to be joyful. You smile as you receive the message. All is well. I am joyful. I am joyful. I am joyful. A joyful energy pulsates throughout your body. You wiggle your fingers and toes. You lie in the yellow crystal sand and move your body around, making snow angels in the crystal sand. It reminds you of when you were a child. You laugh with glee.

To your right, you notice a large yellow crystal the size of a small shed. You are amazed that it is the same shape as the one that was spinning in the air and the ones that were on your body. You realize that the crystal has now enlarged. You run over to the crystal and walk up the angular side of its flat surface. You continue to explore the crystal, just like you were rock climbing. You laugh as you walk around the top of the ridges and down the sides of the crystal. You feel an energy that you have never before experienced, a healing joyful energy. I am joyful. I am joyful. I am full of joy.

A yellow light radiates around you as you stand on one of the crests of the crystal and look across the sparkling yellow crystal beach. I am joyful. I am joyful.

You walk down the side of the crystal and stand at its base. You thank the yellow crystal for the joy you feel throughout your being. (*Pause*)

The sun is glistening across the water as you continue your journey of discovery. You feel a deep sense of joy as your feet sink into the golden sand. You decide that you want to rest and drink in the incredible joy that you feel pulsating throughout your mind and body. You take a deep breath and relax. You feel a deep sense of peace. You close your eyes. All is well. You rest peacefully, better than you have in your whole life. You can feel the healing power of the crystals. Rest and restore. Rest and restore. Rest and restore. (*Pause*)

You sit up, open your eyes and look around. You are still on the same beach, which is now pure white again. Near you, a pale, milky, light green stone lays in the sand. You reach for it and place it in your left hand. As you gaze at it, you notice it is the shape of a house, similar to houses you used to sketch as a child. You can see the sides and the roof, softly rounded, as if it was thatched, but it is crystal. You turn it over and examine the back. It is the same. It feels good in your hand. It starts to warm. You shut your eyes and you feel the energy of the crystal spiralling up your spine. It is a peaceful, safe feeling, and you smile.

You open your eyes and realize that you are now inside the crystal. You feel safe and protected. You lay down on the floor of the crystal. A deep violet colour gently swirls around and through you. You feel the healing power of violet that surrounds you and radiates through you. Then the color turns to a soft pink and swirls around you and through you. Then it becomes a violet and pink with sparkles of silver, like stardust, swirling through the space inside of the crystal. You feel safe and know you are being healed. The healing pink and violet light surrounds you, and you smile.

You take a deep breath and feel thankful for this healing place. (Pause) As you look up, the top of the crystal opens and a brilliant white light fills the space and rests upon you. It is beautiful and energizing. You can feel the healing power. You have a deep inner knowledge that you are being healed, body, mind and spirit. You bask in the oneness that you feel with the white light. Your body is filled with an energy that have never before experienced. You breathe in its essence. You know that you will never forget this place, and the feeling of protection and love. You know that you can come back any time that you wish. "I am healing body, mind and spirit. I am at one with the white light. I am at one with the white light."

You close your eyes and you are once again on the white sand beach. You feel a tremendous sense of gratitude for the experience you have just enjoyed inside the crystal. A warm sun shines down upon you and you feel at peace. (*Pause*)

You open your eyes and notice a bright turquoise object glistening in the white sand. It beckons to you. You lean down to examine it and realize that it is another crystal, beautiful deep turquoise, rectangular in shape. You sit down in the sand and place the crystal in your left hand. You close your eyes, eager to explore the mysteries of this crystal.

You feel the incredible pulsating power of the crystal. The energy goes up your chakras to your head and pulsates back down. It flows down both your arms and out your fingers. It feels like a warm, thick turquoise fluid pulsating through you. Then it goes down your legs and out through your feet. You feel healing as the liquid flows smoothly through your body.

Then you have the sensation that you are swimming in the turquoise liquid. It is warm and comfortable, but you desire to be on land again. You are suddenly transported to a shiny turquoise beach.

You realize that your body has become more fluid and you are covered with a thick turquoise liquid. You can feel it flow around you and through you. You move your head, back, arms and legs, enjoying the feeling of fluidity. You sense a freedom that you have never before experienced. Your body is smooth and flowing. You look toward the ocean and it is turquoise as well. You gaze upwards and, to your amazement, the sky is turquoise.

You hear a message in your mind. You understand that it is meant for you. "You are a part of everything and everything is a part of you. You are perfect and whole, and everything is perfect and whole." (Pause)

You repeat to yourself, "I am a part of everything and everything is a part of me." You smile as the wisdom of the words sink into your soul. "I am perfect and whole, and everything is perfect and whole."

You gaze into the distance of your turquoise world, and see a range of bright golden mountains. The light glistens on the peaks, and you drink in the beauty of the turquoise horizon and the pure golden mountains. You want to explore the golden mountains but understand that this is not the time for you to do that. You breathe deeply into the wonder of the beautiful scene. You know that you will never forget this experience and you will never be the same.

You feel an incredible energy as your whole body tingles with the knowledge of who and what you are. You understand that you are perfect and whole and complete, and connected deeply with everything in the universe. (*Pause*)

You close your eyes. (*Pause*) When you open them, you are once again on the white sand beach. Your heart is full of gratitude for the experience you have had this day and the truths that you have been taught, journeying through the crystals.

Chapter 4   Sleep Enhancement

Sleep Well

by Rosaura Neri

Once upon a time there is a beautiful-minded person who is also dynamic and creative. It is her desire to sleep well through the night.

Her room is full of projects and materials and at night she leaves the new ideas, materials, and projects ready for the next day and gives herself permission to take a rest.

She walks to her resting room...she goes down the stairs...10 steps down...and with every step down...she begins to relax...

10...resting, relax...

9...deep...

8...deeper and deeper...

7...6...sleepy...relax...

5...4...very sleepy...

3...2...deeper and deeper...

1...arriving in the resting room.

This room is the most inviting place to rest and relax...a room free of clutter...containing the perfect bed and mattress for her needs. The walls have the most inviting color to relax, sleep and let go...at her pace...deeper and deeper...relax and let go...

Her body establishes a regular sleep-wake cycle and learns to set its internal clock to her desired schedule. Eventually her clock responds to internal cues to become sleepy at a given time and to awaken at a given time.

Her mind establishes a "winding down" in the evenings...just prior to bedtime and easily becomes free of distracting or troublesome thoughts...ready to engage in a relaxing, enjoyable sleeping time.

A relaxing and enjoyable sleeping time...which continues through the night...pleasant rest...sleep and relax deeply...through the night.

Tomorrow...she will awaken with a refreshed mind...fully rested...new ideas...at the perfect time...a new day.

Sleep like a Baby

by Kelley T. Woods

Anchoring a color that represents relaxation and rest is an easy way to help someone improve their sleep. Although this is a simple process, you can enhance it by using soothing tonality of your voice and allowing for plenty of time for experience and acceptance of the suggestions.

Now that you are feeling so relaxed, so wonderful...make your way to your perfect place...that place deep in your mind that feels safe and comfortable...let me know when you are there...

In your perfect place, there is a sleeping spot. It has the most comfortable bed you can ever imagine and it's waiting for you...go ahead...lie down...your bed feels just like a cloud...as you stretch out on this perfect bed...rest your head on the pillow and look up at the skies...

As you lie there...letting your entire body...from the top of your head to the tips of your toes...become loose... limp...relaxed...just let one thing come into your mind... blue...

Blue...your most favorite shade of blue...a beautiful hue...of blue...blue...blue...let that blue appear right in the middle of your vision...how deep is that blue...how relaxing is that blue...let that blue grow...bigger...deeper...richer...

blue...blue...blue...for you...

All you now can see...or feel...is this wonderful...

peaceful...blue...blue...blue...

Blue...for you...and blue means...you...sleep like a baby...

Let that blue swirl around you...feel it cradle you...perhaps it gently rocks you...

You love blue...blue...blue...

Blue...for you...lets you...sleep like a baby...

Your body is calm...calm like blue...gentle and peaceful...like blue...blue...blue...blue...blue...for you...lets you...sleep like a baby...

Blue...blue...blue...

Big, White, Fluffy Cloud Sleep Inducer

by Susan French

Falling asleep is elusive sometimes, like when you've had very busy or stressful day. If you've ever experienced that, you know how frustrating it can be. If you are one of the unlucky ones, you may have suffered sleep difficulty all of your life. You can be relieved to learn that learning to fall asleep easily and restore a healthy sleeping pattern can be very easy. As the song says: "you just have to know how..."

One thing we've learned about teaching people to return to easy sleep is to suggest that you do not try to calm the mind and the body at the same time. The pattern I'm going to use will alternate: calm the mind, then relax the muscles of the body. By the way, something that I have learned is to tell people to relax their muscles; when you say the general word "relax" to many people, they have no idea how to do that and it's overwhelming. Especially when you are learning how to relax. You start first by relaxing the muscles

One very important part of relaxing mind and body is learning how to breathe in a special way that triggers the release of brain/body tranquillizing neuro-chemicals. If you've ever done yoga, Lamaze for birthing, breathing for relaxation or breathing to play an instrument or to sing, then you probably already know how, but let me go over it in the way I find best.

A good way to take those wonderful, deep yogic-like breath is to pretend that your body is a big balloon and you are going to inflate it with your in-breath (through your nose, preferably), slowly and steadily.

Then hold that breath for just a moment or two, and then slowly and steadily release it until all the breath is gone from your body. Imagine, visualize or pretend that you are blowing away all distractions, all annoyances, all worries or stresses, all tightness in your muscles: left over from the day, all tensions,—blow them all away as you begin to let your empty body balloon collapse like an empty balloon would do. You can easily scan your body if you want to, and let any tight spots become soooo loose that they might feel like jello, or even liquid or even air---that's right.

So let's do some hypnosis to sleep now, as you have learned to do. Make yourself very comfortable. Lie down in a dark, comfortable room, in your comfy bed and simply begin to listen to my soothing, calming voice. There's nothing that you need to do to make this happen or stop it from happening. There is no right way or wrong way. You can begin to let your conscious, alert mind begin to drift off into the background of your mind, as your attention begins to focus inside into your inside awareness. Hypnosis is really a state of inwardly focused awareness. As you listen to my words, your attention is inside, in your ears.

Your inside awareness, often called your subconscious mind, is where all of your memories, thinkings, imaginings, dreams, goals, wishes and wants, and all learning is stored. As you drift deeper into hypnosis or Inside Awareness, you'll find yourself feeling kind of drifty and floaty, as you do when you become lost in thought, or so focused on something, TV, the computer, something you're learning, that anything outside begins to fade out of awareness. That's right. It's so easy, so safe, so natural, so comfortable. You've been listening all this time: see easy and safe it is. So you can simply—relax and listen, even passively, from now on.

It is time to surrender the day. It's gone. It's behind you. Let it drift away into your past for now. And do the same with tomorrow. Tomorrow isn't here yet. It will be here soon enough. But this time is now and this time is for you. You can visualize, imagine or pretend that you are letting yourself become immersed in this wonderful state of "Insideness." And this particular Inside Awareness Time is for you to rest and sleep.

As you allow yourself to drift into this wonderful Inside Awareness we call hypnosis, let me suggest several things to you that will help you to go as deeply into this state as you wish.

Each and every time you hear me say the words deep, deeper, or deeply down, let this be a reminder to you to let go and drift. When I say the words relax, drifty or drowsy, let yourself do that. It's just a reminder to let go a little more.

In fact, as you find yourself drifting down, a little more at a time, you might find yourself wondering if it the sound of my voice that seems to pull you gently down deeper. Or is it the words that I saw that just make you want to sink even more deeply down? Or you might even notice that there is a tendency for you to drift even more deeply down in the little pauses and silences between my words. It's that easy.

It is time now for wonderful, restful sleep in which you can crowd out all thoughts of both yesterday AND tomorrow. This time is for you. This is your time to let all things fade away into the darkness and let yourself drift into wonderful, calming, sleeping rest.

Your mind might even let your thoughts drift back to some time in your past when you were so sleepy and tired you were at the threshold of sleep before you know it. And before you knew it, you drifted behind the veil of sleep, and into wonderful dreams and the bliss of sweet and darkened sleep. That's right.

If you can remember exactly what it was like when you were so close to falling behind the veil of sleep, you might even find yourself slipping past the threshold and drifting off without even remembering and that's perfectly perfect, isn't it?

(*pause for a few moments*)

But if you haven't done that yet, slipped and drifted off into wonderful, beautiful, restful sleep, let's go back to breathing and follow your breathing cycle again.

Can you soften and loosen those eyelids? Twice as much more relaxed if you can? Relax all the tiny muscles around your eyes. How good it feels to do this. Make certain that the little space between your eyebrows are smooth and without furrows. And your forehead, let it be as smooth and relaxed as the forehead of a baby as it falls asleep. Or a pet. Or a child. Or your mate. That's right. It can be easily, just because you think it, those wonderful waves of pure, loose, letting go of all muscles, can't help but let go...that's right.

And then let those wonderful, perfectly temperatured waves of sleepiness and relaxation flow from the top of your head, down and around, and even through your body, loosen your tummy muscles, down into your hips, thighs, knees and all the way down to your tippy toes.

You might take a moment to notice if your toes are warm and relaxed as you relax more and more, or do they feel cool or even numb, as if they aren't even there. You might even begin to notice that you feel as if you are all brain and consciousness with no body awareness at all. However you experience this relaxation and letting go is perfectly perfect for you, isn't' it?

And so now we begin to let go of the day to drift off into the wonderful, drifty, drowsiness of peaceful, quiet sleep. Are you ready now? Or will you be more ready to drift away in a moment or two, when you're more ready? It's up to you of course. And it doesn't really matter because you are half-way asleep already, if not more. You might even be more than half-way asleep. It doesn't matter at all, does it?

Sometimes it is just too hard to relax the busy mind chatter and relax the body at the same time, so we can break it up.

Let's calm the mind first. First, can you imagine big, white, fluffy clouds crowding your busy mind so much that it crowds out all room for anything else, and your mind can begin to become quiet and still, can't it? Because when you're imagining beautiful, fluffy white clouds, still or floating, whatever you prefer, there simply is no room for mind chatter.

And so you notice a tendency for your body to relax while you do this. In fact, if you took a wonderful, yogic, sleepy breath, before you imagined the clouds, you'll notice even more of a tendency for your body to—relax---release—let go. Becoming softer and looser and floatier and driftier—that's right.

You know that it's perfectly perfect to lose track of course.

The more you lose track of where you are in the process the better. And your body lets go even looser and sleepier. And your mind becomes more and more still and quiet. As still and quiet as a pool of water that is so still it is like a pane of glass. That's right.

And then you think of the clouds again. And you fill up your mind with big, white fluffy clouds again. So full that no thoughts can come in. That's right.

But if a thought manages to drift into your mind, simply notice it. And then release your attention to that thought. Watch it drift off into the darkness, or into the white, fluffy cloud, and you watch until it fades to nothing, nothing, nothing.

Then easily bring your attention back to your breathing; take another deep, yogic sleep-inducing breath, and notice how your mind and body relax even more, as your sense of trance, and sleep, seem to deepen, all by themselves. That's right. Letting go, even more.

And you can continue this simple pattern until you fall off to sleep.

However, if you're having one of those really bad nights, and sleep has not whisked you away by now, you can add one more thing. You can imagine that you are staring at those big, fluffy clouds and you can notice that the number 300 is printed on it. It can be a number or it can be writing. You could even start at a 1000 if you wish. It doesn't matter because you'll be asleep long before you get anywhere at all.

Whatever number you've picked, see that number across the white, fluffy cloud. Watch it as it fades away, up off into darkness or into the cloud, until it fades away to nothing, nothing, nothing.

Take another nice, easy, relaxing breath, let all muscles go loose, smooth, heavy, sleepy, relaxed, and begin again with the next big, white, fluffy cloud with the number 299 on it and do the same thing.

Remember to watch the number fade away. Bring your attention easily back to your breath. Then send the relaxing message to all of your muscles. Take a moment to make sure that they have indeed loosened up a little more. You might even well be drifting off into hypnosis, which is the gateway to sleep.

And then you come back to your clouds. Don't be a bit surprised if you begin to forget to remember the numbers you have just counted, or the number you're supposed to count next. It's good to forget. It's good to forget to remember or to remember to forget. We forget things all the time, don't we?

They just float away into nothing like a thousand of little pieces of paper. Kind of like when you forget what you had for breakfast, 3 weeks ago on Wednesday or who called you closest to noon, two weeks ago on Monday. It's unimportant. We just forget, don't we?

Like when you have a word on the tip of your tongue and the harder you try to remember, the more forgotten it becomes. Or when you walk into a room and you can't for the life of you remember what you went in there to do. And the harder you try to remember, the more forgotten it becomes.

So should you forget the number you've just counted, or the

next number you're supposed to count, or if it is time to relax your muscles or to take a good deep breath, it doesn't matter at all, does it? You just pick a spot to continue. You just guess or make it up. Because nothing matters more than you drifting off to wonderful, peaceful, quiet, restful sleep. That's right, isn't? Of course it is? It couldn't be righter.

And I'll bet by the time you get to this part, you'll be sound, sound asleep. And even if you haven't drifted off completely, this level of relaxation of both mind and body, will give you more rest certainly, than worrying or tossing or turning on the computer or TV which as stimulants, will just wake you up even more.

Actually, if you get bored or you're not yet asleep, you can imagine anything drifting off into the sky: colors, balloons, hats, papers, people you don't like, or people you are mad at, or whatever. And each time you do THAT, remember to let it fade and come easily back to your breathing...and letting go...softer, looser, sleepier, closer and closer to the threshold of sweet, deep, dark, restful sleeping and even dreaming.

Sweet, sweet dreams, precious dreamer. Sweet, sweet dreams.

Chapter 5   Hypnotic Poetry

Healing with the Use of Poetry

by Janice Lesley

Background: My underlying philosophy was to stop defending myself when I became cognizant of an irrational sense of panic arising when confronted with very specific events. I would first attempt to find a way to stay with the feelings of panic and then see what lay behind my thoughts and feelings attached to the panic.

Then I wanted to express my experience in the form of a poem. In order to do this I allowed myself some time to specifically invite and welcome the 'dreaded feelings of panic' - which is when I experienced a surprising result.

My Innocence Returned

I let the panic come.
But, this time I found *a way to stay.*
I didn't move as
it washed over me,
a tsunami of emotion.

This once,
I did not keep busy,
defending myself
against my thoughts
of what I called, "Panic".

Instead, I found myself set free.
The thoughts no more

....than thoughts
rendered harmless,
their effects, no more.

It was then that I felt
something coming.
A treasure,
being revealed...
A presence emerging.

Pale translucent,
she once hid.
The colors of night
all around her embedded
in shades of darkest blue.

"Hello", I said softly
as she looked at me.
"You are beautiful", I said,
so innocent and pure.

You are that part of me
which left in fear.
And all this time,
when I felt the panic
I had run, too.

I never once imagined
how you were hidden
beneath it.
Your gentle presence,
awaiting in the dark.

A little willingness
to change my mind
released and rescued
us both in time.
I found you!   My Innocence Returned

Never Too Late

by Doris Santic

Never too late to be whom you want to be.
Never too late to change your thoughts, beliefs, and perceptions.
Never too late to be optimistic, enthusiastic, and happy!
Never too late to have a great attitude.
Never too late to be more adaptable in every situation.
Never too late to embrace unavoidable change, rather than fight it.
Never too late to forgive yourself and others.
Never too late to learn and grow and be good to ourselves along the way.
Never too late to get unstuck.

Never too late to change our ways and try new things.
Never too late to expand your mind and believe your perceptions equal your reality.
Never too late to incorporate a sense of humor in all things which happen around us.
Never too late to see the good in everything!
Never too late to remember that every obstacle you meet in life can be seen as a block or an opportunity.
Never too late to learn from our mistakes and failures, they are just signs of what did not work for us.
Never too late to listen to and get to know your children.
Never too late to fill your heart with love for yourself and others, including strangers and animals.

Never too late to be fun and adventurous and feel excited about life.
Never too late to make new friends to enjoy, who support your true self.
Never too late to heal yourself from all the hurt and pain.
Never too late to laugh out loud at least once a day.

Never too late to heal old wounds and enjoy life to the fullest.
Never too late to be a survivor who loves surviving.
Never too late to accomplish those dreams and desires that
were your first love.
Never too late to feel every good emotion you ever want to
feel.
Never too late to feel sexy and beautiful and celebrate your
uniqueness.
Never too late to let go of the past, not worry about the
future, instead learn to live and enjoy the present moment.

Never too late to love yourself truly so that you won't need
approval from others.
Never too late to live up to your own expectations.
Never too late to be a best friend to yourself first.
Never too late to think outside your box and be open to new
ideas.
Never too late to bring balance to work and play.
Never too late to enjoy sex and be more playful.
Never too late to live freely in every way possible.
Never too late to be the best you, you can be!
Never too late to feel this life has all been worth it as you
continue to learn and grow.

Never too late to want the best for yourself and think
thoughts with no limitations.
Never too late to dream big and know that you deserve it!
Never too late to focus on the good instead of the bad.
Never too late to learn fear has no place in our minds and
our hearts.
Never too late to know true love which can be found through
work or relationships.
Never too late to use our minds and imagination to create
our lives.
Never too late to know and understand we are all connected.
Never too late to pay attention and be aware of ourselves.

Never too late to get the most out of life and truly experience feelings of happiness for no reason at all.
Never too late to appreciate and be grateful for everything.
Never too late to feel truly loved and appreciated.
Never too late to release any guilt, anger, or resentments in our body and mind.
Never too late to let go of anything that does not align with your higher self.
Never too late to go after what you really want in life!
Never too late to say those things you've always wanted to say.
Never too late to see the beauty in the world and beauty in others.
Never too late to fill our hearts with love until they overflow with joy.

Never too late to be true to yourself now and always.
Never too late to live by your own rules for your own wants.
Never too late to truly learn to enjoy all the lessons of the world we live in.
Never too late to live your life with no regrets.
Never too late for a new beginning.
Never too late to always focus on the end result, which is what you want!

There's still time to be whole...the sooner you start, the longer you have to enjoy the outcome!

The Eyes of Ellis Island

by Joanna Cameron

Hat pins, knitting needles, hampers, trunks,
Hats, rumpled shirts, lace, cutlery and china
Artifacts of people's lives
As they leave their native country behind
For a necessary reason
Making a difficult decision
To do the right thing

And now what to pack
On such a journey
Taking what's important to you
To take care of yourself
To take care of your young
Taking just a few things
Needed for a new life
In a different country

Pictures in black and white of exhausted people
Tired faces, questioning eyes
Focused eyes filled with expectation
Eyes that say - I don't understand

What's next
A railway ticket to meet a relative in the
Midwest, perhaps
Stressed eyes that question
Will I pass the physical
Will I receive a stamp of approval
Will the Statue of Liberty deliver for me

Moving through the process
To a new life in a free country
And what is it that moves people

From one place to another
Something changing within
The same change that moves
Wildebeest across the tundra
Salmon up the river
Whales to the south
Turtles to the same beach
Where they were born
Because change is instinctual
Change is inevitable
Something stirring within

And it was pictures of California
Orange trees, the ocean, the mountains
People skiing and surfing
That moved this British schoolgirl
To make a decision
To go to California
And finally to be an American
And our daughter as a little girl
Doodled palm trees everywhere
Miniature flip flops dangle from the car mirror
And so she made a decision
A move to a college in the south
To challenge herself

And I wonder as I often do
What moves you
What is your compelling future
Now, this student is a teacher
And remains a student
And what will you see I wonder
As you look into the mirror
Six months from now
A healthy body with new behaviors

YOU

And when you started your journey with me
You wondered
What is the best way to
Let go of the weight
Stop overeating
And to your surprise you found that
You forgot about food
Your life is full with other activities and interests
You are healthy

And when you think of that person
That you said you always wanted to be
That you could be
And then you realize
That you ARE that person

NOW

Aren't you

Chapter 6   Ego-Strengthening

Words of Wisdom

by Lani Nicholls

In this age and stage of my life, as an Elder, walking this earth path for the past 73 years, (yes, I walked before the age of 1), I share the following as my way of giving back and supporting you on your life's journey.

In our minds, that deep wellspring of wisdom within, we seek solace. We talk to ourselves, wonder about things, question, consider, create, and make choices. We give shape and substance to our lives through the choices we make. For me, it was one of those choices that lead me here, to this present moment, sharing these words with you.

As a professional hypnotherapist for close to 30 years, I've been thinking about what words of wisdom I could share with those remarkable women who are giving new life to this profession. Trusting my knowing, my mind carried me back to my early training with my teacher-mentor and friend, Charles Tebbetts. I've always remembered something Charles shared about working with people, especially in a situation that made you feel uncomfortable..."*If you were born in that person's body, and experienced everything that person experienced, at the same age, you would be exactly like them.*" (Note, the key words here are *at the same age-*think about it.)

So, one word of wisdom to pass on is COMPASSION. Remember to be compassionate with yourself. You do have compassion, otherwise, you would not be doing this work.

My knowing tells me that we do not choose this work, this work chooses us. We are called to it in different ways...often because of something happening in one's life or with someone we are close to. The call is not what's important, what's important is that you had the courage to answer the call. So, another word on the wisdom list is COURAGE. Acknowledge your courage.

You have chosen to become a pioneer...a pioneer exploring and expanding the inner workings of the mind. Quantum science, brain and mind research, neuro-plasticity; so many frontiers are expanding the knowledge base we have available to develop our skills, and there is so much more to come. Your courage to pursue a road-less-traveled, *hypnosis*, contributes to that expanding knowledge, bringing a better understanding in this emerging field of healing.

Coming to mind now is the word, CONNECTION, taking its place on the list. Connection can be defined as something that "connects" or brings together two or more things. As hypnotic women, we help people resolve inner conflict that leads to distress by helping those we work with gain awareness and connect (or re-connect) their conscious choices with their subconscious beliefs in empowering ways. Our connections with others, our colleagues, our family, our friends help us grow and flourish as well as providing us with the means and opportunities to help make our world a better place.

Speaking of connection as "something that connects one or more things," for me that something is SPIRIT. Many people talk about wanting to follow a spiritual path, or being on a spiritual path. My knowing, for me, is that my life is my spiritual path...it is not something separate from me. It is what called me to this work when I was just a child. Whatever your beliefs, whatever sustains you and gives you strength to live each day, Spirit or spirituality is for you to define. I am simply sharing something of my spiritual path and how it relates to my work as a hypnotic woman. For me,

Spiritual Connection is what has guided me through all the twists and turns my life has taken. If you so choose, Spiritual Connection can take its place on the list.

I spoke of being called to this work and I want to share some of my personal story but before I do, I want you to know I do so with the intention that something in my words may be meaningful or helpful to you in some way. Sometimes we are touched by something and the effect of it is not immediate but at another point in time its memory arises and we have one of those Ah-Ha moments.

I just had an Ah-Ha moment, so I'll jump to that moment, the memory of a story...a true story, shared with me many years ago when I was working with Native American youth. I do so as a way to show the importance of the words of wisdom we have on our list so far.

> Alan, a teenage boy, was standing next to a tree talking on his phone. He noticed another teenage boy (Richard) across the street, a person who he had seen at school, cleaning out his locker but had never before spoken to.
>
> As Alan watched the other boy, he noticed he was struggling to carry a load of books and things, dropping them and having trouble picking them up. Alan felt a sense of *compassion,* he wanted to help but Alan was very shy, reluctant to approach someone he didn't know. Moved by Richard's struggle, he found the *courage* to cross the street and say, "Hi, I'm Alan...need a hand?"
>
> Richard looked startled and afraid but then *honored* Alan's offer and said, "Sure, man, thanks!" As they walked along they realized they lived only a block apart and had some of the same interests. Arriving home, Richard thanked Alan for the help. Something stirred in Alan and, without thinking, he gave Richard

his phone number (*connection*) and said, "Call me if you want to hang out." Alan thought he saw a tear in Richard's eye as he walked away.

What Alan didn't know was that Richard was feeling hopeless and powerless, lonely and afraid, neglected by his alcoholic mother and absent father. Feeling like he was worthless, he cleaned out his locker and planned to go home and commit suicide.

That brief connection between the two boys made a real difference. Richard was touched by a glimmer of hope, so he decided not to go ahead with his plan. We never know how our actions will affect another person. Sometimes, just a passing hello or a smile is enough to make a real difference in someone's life.

Another word that comes to mind is HONOR. When we honor something, we acknowledge it, respect it. When you are gifted with something, honor it by saying "yes" to it. When we refuse a gift, whatever form it takes, we dishonor it by saying no. Think of a time you were gifted with a compliment and felt uncomfortable receiving it. Not accepting diminishes the giver, not the gift. Honor your own gifts, whatever they may be. Like they say in Native country, *"The Honor of One is the Honor of All."*

"The Farther Back You Can Look, the Farther Forward You Can See."

Somewhere in my past, when I first read that quote from Winston Churchill, it struck a chord inside me and from time to time it floats across my mind, bringing with it thoughts about influences that have shaped my life as a hypnotic woman.

INFLUENCES...another word for the list. Your life, your experience, whatever that may be, influences and gives shape

144

and substance to the work you do as a hypnotist:

I mentioned earlier that I was called to this work at a young age. I've always felt different...I didn't fit the molds that everyone else seemed to. I was a child, yet I had knowings and saw things no one else did. My mother was always making the sign of the cross and telling me "You shouldn't know such things." I was like my mother; she knew what would happen before it did, but she was afraid to acknowledge it. As a child I didn't understand that I was highly intuitive, what some call *clair-cognizant*. My saving grace was my Native American father who would just look at me and smile a knowing smile, and without a word, I knew that he knew and I was okay. INTUITION is part of my heritage so it takes a special place on the list for me.

I remember when I was 7 years old, looking at my mother and the words jumped out of my mouth, "When I grow up I'm going to look into people's minds, say the right words and help them be happy." My mother had a shocked look on her face, made the sign of the cross, twice this time, and just looked at me without a word. I went outside, climbed up my favorite tree and that was it, the veil of forgetfulness clouded the memory. I did not understand until many years later the influence those words would have on my life.

Fast forward to 1985. When I stepped across the threshold for the first time of the Charles Tebbetts Hypnotism Training Institute in Edmonds WA, I felt a shift inside. My intention had been to get information about self-hypnosis to deal with the stress of taking care of my mother who had Alzheimer's disease. Little did I realize I would be sitting in on Charlie's live class. Sitting there, I knew this was where I was meant to be and this was the work I was here to do...I didn't know how, I just knew I would. I became certified as a Hypnotherapist, a Clinical Hypnotherapist and then I was honored by Charles when he asked me to become one of his Certified Hypnotism Instructors, saying "yes!" without hesitation.

When I opened my first private practice, the public knew very little about hypnosis, so educating the public about it was important to me. I had given a presentation for an organization and later that day I received a call from a woman who told me a friend had heard my presentation and thought it was fascinating and she wanted to know if I made house calls. I told her I did, but I would first need to schedule a consultation. She agreed and came into the office, and in a very demanding way, she offered to pay me double my fee if I would come to her home that evening. She wanted me to hypnotize her husband so she could ask him questions about what he had been up to, because she knew he had been up to something and he refused to talk to her about it.

I took a deep breath, exhaled and told her, "That is not how I work. I am a professional hypnotherapist, and that would be highly unethical, something I would not do. If your husband asked me to do hypnosis with him, that would be different." She offered me more money and I refused. I offered to give her a sample session but she made a grumbling sound, got up and slammed my door on the way out. I had to laugh to myself, like some cosmic joke had just been played. Another word for our list...INTEGRITY, whatever that means to you.

All things begin and end, so it's time to wrap it up, as they say. And so, I leave you with the beginning of your own list of words of wisdom, to add to and pass on in your own way:

Compassion   Courage   Connection Spiritual Connection
Honor   Influences   Intuition   Integrity

I leave you with my Give Away...a tool of sorts that I created several years ago for my own self-care, becoming a tool I still use with clients and in groups...I call it my *Spirit Box*. (Note, make it your own...call it what you will. It's about the essence, not the name.)

First, I took some blank index cards (any size you want) and wrote words, thoughts, affirmations, quotes, whatever came to mind. You can begin with the words we have just explored.

I began with a basket and later found a special box to put the cards in. As I began my day, I would reach into the box and pull out a card. Whatever was on the card became my focus for my day. I trusted my intuition to guide me so whatever card I drew was always *right on* for me.

I created some cards, words or affirmations I often used in sessions, having the client draw a card to use as homework, serving as thought triggers for practicing their self-hypnosis or meditation. Clients often told me they found it both helpful and meaningful for them. This can be done individually or in groups.

I've utilized this process in women's groups I've led. At the beginning of the group I gave each person an index card and had them write down a topic, question or issue they wanted to explore and learn more about as part of our group. I would then have someone draw a card and that would become our focus. What was interesting was that I would prepare something in advance along with handouts, and they would always be in sync...just what was needed for the card that was pulled for that session. Coincidence is not my belief. Again, for me, trusting my intuition always works best.

The subconscious mind is the feminine mind, the seat of our emotions...the well spring of our creativity and intuition. Tap into your feminine mind and have the courage to think outside the box in your approach to your work. The mind is powerful, the body knows how to heal itself and when they work together, it's a joyful experience. Lighten up and enjoy being a hypnotic woman.

With Love & Light, *Lani*

Archetype Alignment

by Kelley T. Woods

Each of us have many different aspects to our personalities ...some of them are more obvious, such as the part of us that is the child of our parent or perhaps the brother or sister to a sibling or maybe even a parent to our child...there is a part of us which yearns at times to be a partner to someone special, in a romantic way or via a more plutonic connection. We may also be aware of the student part of us, the productive, income-earning part of us or the part of us which loves to engage in sport or physical activity.

These parts, or ego states, exist within us all, to some degree, and they help us navigate through our lives. We may be aware when we are assuming certain identities in a stronger sense, and subduing others.

When we are feeling balanced and healthy, the various aspects of our personalities are working in congruence and we find it smooth sailing through life. But, when we are struggling, especially with forces of inner conflict, these characters are no longer in alignment.

It is desirable to become aware not only of the many tones of yourself, but to become aware of how they work for you. This experience is designed to introduce you to some very special aspects of your personality, to give you a chance to learn how they influence and help you, and to establish a deeper relationship with them.

It is my objective to be your tour guide here, not to dictate who or what you should be, but to allow you to discover some wonderful innate qualities of yourself which have always been, and will continue to be, within you.

Following induction and deepener:

Imagine, now, a meeting place of some type. It might be a large table surrounded by comfortable chairs, it could be an open fire pit with log seating, or perhaps it's a round stone hovering in midair...whatever you prefer is just right for you. Notice that there is a special place for you to sit; it's the place of command and you make yourself comfortable there now.

I'd like you to begin with summoning forth a part of yourself that you are already familiar with; this is the part of you that represents your strength and your ability to take action. We might think of this aspect of yourself as the Warrior, or perhaps you think of it as the Fighter, or the Protector...or the Hero. You know that this part was present at times in your past when you were feeling a sense of determination, when you were creating the emotional commitment you needed to do whatever you needed to do.

Invite this Inner Warrior to join you in this setting now...and take some time to notice everything about this powerful and focused part of your personality. Notice how your Warrior manifests physically: the shape, the features, any dress or accoutrements, tools or even, weapons.

And now, begin to feel a deep bond beginning to form between you and this formidable champion...let a feeling of trust flow between you as you relay your appreciation and gratitude for all that your Warrior does for you. Your Warrior's ultimate goal is your happiness and success and you can take some time now to reflect on how this part of you

149

plays an important role in your life.

(pause)

Next, please invite a part of you that is very special. This part of you represents your intuition, your humor, your imagination. It's been described as the Magician, or the Fairy Godmother, or the Maverick...even the Wise Guy!

The ability to tell the silent truth about a situation helps the Magician to find solutions; and this gift often arrives as if by a snap of the fingers or a kiss blown in the air. Your Magician can solve things in an instant, using whimsy and humor...because it's all magic – invisible and ethereal.

Pay close attention as your Magician appears and joins you. This is a part of you which can detach from anything, just sitting to the side, observing it. It may even decide to sit on top of the table, or beneath it! Your Magician is sometimes irreverent, always creative and humorous. Notice how this part manifests physically: the shape, the features, any dress or accoutrements, tools or even, toys.

Take some time now and get to know your Magician...establish a light-hearted connection with this part of your personality that loves to help you through laughter and play and intuition. Your Magician's ultimate goal is your happiness and you can take some time now to reflect on how this part of you plays an important role in your life.

(pause)

Now, it's time to invite a wonderful part of you to this gathering. I'd like you to meet the aspect of your personality which signifies your deepest emotional connection to others and to the world itself. This is the part of you which we might call the Lover, or the Loving One. You may also think of it as the Caretaker or the Protector.

The Loving One inside of you is the source of your feeling of connection and compassion for others. The Loving One is the epitome of unconditional love, unconditional acceptance...

...not just for others, but for yourself. This is the deepest essence of love and is the purest part of who you are.

We are all born with this Loving One and it dwells within us, looking for opportunity to express that innate, rich and satisfying experience of loving unconditionally. Let your Loving One shine as it joins you here now...see it in all of its glory, all of its brilliance. Notice how this aspect of yourself manifests physically: the shape, the features, any dress or accoutrements, gifts or symbols.

How will you know when your Loving One is working for you, when it is present? Notice the ways...perhaps with a warm hug, a compassionate whisper...a patient smile? Let the awareness of how your Loving One works for you imbed itself deep in your mind.

(pause)

Please, consider now a part of yourself which can be described as the Sovereign. This aspect resembles a King or a Queen and holds a position of power and ultimate wisdom. Your Sovereign is just and fair and is a source of your personal integrity. As the senior part of this group, it also holds authority over the others and can intercede, dictate and govern on your behalf.

Notice how this aspect of yourself manifests physically: the shape, the features, any dress or accoutrements, gifts or

151

symbols. Spend some time getting to know your King or Queen now...

How will you know when your Sovereign is working for you, when it is present? Notice the ways...perhaps with a wise decision, perhaps with compromise, or maybe by showing you your moral compass? Let the timeless knowledge of how your Sovereign works for you imbed itself deep in your mind.

(pause)

Will you now, please, turn your attention to the spirit of cooperation between all these aspects of yourself?...you might notice how they are balanced or represented to you... Does one of these characters exert more influence than another? Observe how they all work together, or perhaps they haven't been working together very well at all...whatever you notice, I want you to realize that you are in the position of power here; you are the most important one and you are the one in control.

Imagine now that you can adjust anything that needs adjusting, as simply as waving a hand gently in the air and guiding them all toward a balanced point. Maybe you want to adjust the height of the chairs or seats...or blow a kiss to change the light that illuminates each of your parts...

You don't have to think about the details of this; just trust that your dynamic subconscious mind knows how to do this. Take a wonderful, energizing breath...and as you exhale, feel everything fall into place...naturally...perfectly...for you.
Please also observe that these various aspects of your personality enjoy this balancing...and that this draws their attention toward each other, so that they now fully appreciate the value of working together, in congruence for your wishes and desires. See that connection of agreement manifesting now...feel the camaraderie; the love that they share...with you as their common link.

152

(pause)

If there is a particular goal that you are desiring in your life...imagine placing that request before you right now...it may be represented by a tangible item, or a word or even just a thought. Just place it out there and ask your personality aspects to help you with this...each one has a way to assist you and will now work independently, yet also as a team to move you toward this goal...this dream...
Thank them; show your gratitude and appreciation for all that they do for you...and when you are ready, let them assimilate back into yourself, where they will now support you in an enhanced endeavor to let you live a happier and healthier life.

Take another, wonderful and deep energizing breath...and as you exhale...let yourself imagine all of the marvelous possibilities that are coming to you as a result of this experience. You will find that from this point forward, you will become more aware of how each aspect of your personality is positively influencing you at certain times...*and*...you will realize that you can call forth specific ones to help you when you need them...

Facilitating a Spirit Journey

by Mary Lee LaBay

A modified version of a journey, combining traditional techniques with hypnosis, is as follows: The client prepares by relaxing in a comfortable position. Begin by using your preferred induction and deepening. You may use a rattle or drum, or play relaxing music.

Imagine that you are standing in a clearing in the forest. Tall trees stand all around you, and a shaft of light pours down on this clearing through an opening in the trees. Feel the warmth of the sunlight. Notice the scent of the forest, as you relax deeper and deeper into this scene.

Guides and helpers have come to support your journey today, and they gather all around you. To your right you notice your male guides, ancestors, totems, animals, and objects. As you look to the right, who and what do you notice?

To your left are your female guides, ancestors, totems, animals, and objects. As you look to the left, who and what do you notice?

Your guides and helpers lead you now along a path through the woods to the edge of a body of water. What do you notice about this body of water? Is it a river, a lake, or an ocean? Do you notice anything else?

Along the bank is a birch bark canoe. Your guides invite you to get into the canoe, and one of the guides joins you there. Who is the guide that will accompany you on your journey?

Behind you is an object that has been placed there for your protection. What do you know about that object of protection?

The canoe moves away from the bank and begins to move on the water. What do you notice next?

From here continue to ask non-leading questions to reveal any messages, lessons, discoveries, or adventures that they have on their journey. Continue on with curiosity about their journey until it appears that they have gotten the messages they were to receive. Then, gently guide them back to the bank of the body of water where they can get out of the canoe.

On land, they can reunite with their guides to exchange any further messages, and they can show their gratitude for the guidance and support.

Take some time to go over the story, discussing what the client has learned and how they will integrate that material into their daily lives.

If there are parts of the story that present a negative or challenging experience, you can ask the client to go back through the story, in the trance state, and allow the subconscious mind to revise it in a way that turns out more favorably. Then, discuss how they would make correlating changes in their behaviors or choices to likewise improve their life.

End the session by bringing them out of the trance state in the way that you choose.

Modification:

As stated above, it is sometimes wise to have the client envision the journey as a walk on a path. Simply ask them to envision walking on a path, and have them describe what that path looks like. Then, continue with non-leading questions through the journey to the end.

Your Beautiful Container

by Carole Fawcett

Suggested script for women with either visible or non-visible disabilities or women who have self esteem issues due to body image. This can be adapted for any age, any disability (use of mobility aids, use of wheelchairs). The key to the wording is to always put the person before the disability or the mobility aid; i.e.: Person with M.S.; Person who uses a wheelchair – as opposed to Person IN a wheelchair.

As you continue to become one with the calmness, the tranquility and the serenity of your surroundings, visualize yourself as being a beautiful loving soul. Feel the peaceful serenity of that knowledge as it washes over you. Imagine that you are standing in a large, well lit dressing room with two floor-to-ceiling mirrors.

In your mind. see yourself wearing a beautiful silk kimono, patterned with dainty pink and white roses. You are feeling so pretty and feminine as you visualize this. Really see this in your mind's eye. Imagine, too, that your favourite scent is in the air as well. Ahh...it soothes your senses and you feel very safe and secure.

You turn around slowly, facing the mirror...you let the gown slide off your shoulders and drop to the floor, looking at the reflection of yourself in the mirror. As you begin to focus on your perceived flaws, something stops you and you feel and sense a wonderful change in your perception of yourself. You feel a sense of love and acceptance wash over you as you reflect upon your own image. You are feeling loved just the way you are.

You know that you are a good person, a kind person, a generous person and a very caring person. You know that your body is simply a container for all the goodness that is in your soul. The container may not be as perfect as you would like it to be, but inside it is full of wonderfully important things. Feel gratitude for the wonderfulness of you.

See yourself filling your container up with positive feelings and thoughts about yourself. Gently place 'kindness' into the container, followed by 'thoughtfulness' and then 'confidence' and 'pride'. Take a moment to really think about all the positives that you hold inside your personal container...be very honest and open with yourself. It is okay to acknowledge your own goodness, in fact you must do this to honour who you are.

See past your idea of imperfection in your own image, allow room for tenderness towards yourself...knowing that nobody is perfect in any way. That makes everyone as perfect as they individually can be. This includes you. Allow that thought and that belief to empower you. Really believe this.

See yourself standing in front of the mirror in the dressing room and say to your image "I Love You Just The Way You Are". Say this to yourself every day. Feel the love wash over you.

You are an amazing and beautiful soul and you will start to recognize this and feel much better about yourself every day.

Finding Love Within

by Camilla Edborg

I usually use this script in sections, taking one part per session. Start after desired level of relaxation.

Allow yourself to simply relax and follow my voice and we will go on an amazing journey to find something helpful and lovely thing about yourself that you didn't know. Imagine you are walking down some beautiful stairs down to a garden...this garden has a secret door that helps you come to your inner self. So see this beautiful door, and you know there is something to look forward to...so simply open this door go through and gently close it.

Imagine yourself walking on a beautiful path, feeling absolutely wonderful, relaxed and safe. You can notice the flowers, bushes and trees in the background, the scent is the way you like it, the breeze and sun is just perfect. Butterflies and other animals you like are around, friendly to you and each other...Everything is peaceful and in harmony.

Part 1

The path leads you to a little pond...one of those wonderful ponds where you can see clearly down to the bottom. Some small colorful fishes are curious and if you want to, you can put your hand in the water and let them touch your hand gently...it tickles sometimes...the colors are clear, sky is fantastic...yes - it is a perfect day.

Sometimes you can find personal messages that are meant for you in the bottom of the clear water...in the sand... messages that your inner self wants you to notice to help you. So let's see if there is a message..let your gaze relax and see if there is a message.

Does it say anything? *(write this down...sometimes it's nothing, then just keep moving)*

You can simply walk slowly and enjoy this walk until you reach a beautiful, big, wise tree. The funniest thing is, that on the stem there is a magic mirror. Let's go there and have a look. Look into the mirror now, can you see yourself? Describe what you see... *(also to check their critical issues)*

Take this opportunity to look at yourself...at your whole body. How does it feel?

(usually not too positive; very critical...write this down to work on later)

Let's look properly, more closely this time, not the shell, because there is something pretty amazing you need to see and it's hidden. Now let the body almost become see-through, and unimportant...like it is a temporary shell, let's look what lovely thing there is INSIDE...

I now ask you to look inside and find that person...that person who has gone through so much, learnt so much, tried so hard...loved and had losses...and yet is standing here, in such a beautiful way.

Describe what you feel and see?

(Write this down and share with client when fully awake, can also be used later as a reminder, also set in different scripts and ways to help client. The goal is to help the client see the wonderful part inside of her, focus on the beauty inside, be proud and to appreciate who he/she is, and to love oneself - flaws and all, and to strive to be better in their own pace. To see that the body is something there to HELP

the client so the goal is to be appreciative and start liking the body/appearance too)

Look closer...look at the eyes... see it's almost like a universe. How beautiful. Find the core of that beautiful inner YOU and you can start to appreciate everything you have been through in this journey called Life. All the experiences you have made and grown so many insights and wisdom from...look and appreciate...look and feel the wonderful feeling growing, and growing...and when you really look, appreciate and see your core, there is no need to be harsh on yourself, instead, look inside and love yourself for trying, love yourself for all the things in life you go through...just simply love...appreciate and love YOU!

Look at yourself with new eyes and appreciate ...and love...You are beautiful inside. You glow...You are unique and wonderful just the way you are. You will naturally keep growing and gaining new insights - How amazing is that?
Just let the feeling grow...Can you feel it?

Now take a deep breath and forgive YOURSELF...You have been too critical of yourself...forgive yourself, because you didn't know better. You didn't have the tools to understand properly. Forgive yourself and feel FREE...absolutely free. Deep in your heart, find the way and forgive yourself truly...

(wait a moment... see if client has truly forgiven, as this helps very much in process)

From now on you can appreciate yourself more, be able to give yourself some special time of peace of mind...and enjoy feeling good inside...always remembering the lovely feeling of seeing the true you in a grateful and loving way.

We thank the tree for showing us this useful and great insight. When you are ready, let's walk back to the pond.

161

Let's check again if anything is written in the sand...what does it say?

Slowly and very harmoniously, take your time to walk back...feeling absolutely wonderful, finding the door out, closing it after yourself, enjoying your new insights so much more. Positive feelings are filling your whole body...you are feeling great and in a moment, when you are ready, come back to here and now, keeping these wonderful feelings.

(*Go through the letters written in the sand [if any]. These are very useful insights and usually help the client with what he/she is going through.*)

Part 2

Allow yourself to simply relax and follow my voice and we will go on an amazing journey to find something helpful and lovely thing about you that you didn't know.

Imagine yourself walking on a beautiful path, feeling absolutely wonderful, relaxed and safe. You can notice the flowers, bushes and trees in the background, the scent is the way you like it, the breeze and sun is just perfect. Everything is peaceful and in harmony.

Let's walk just a little bit further...enjoy just walking and feeling wonderful after all these insights...the weather is just the way you like it...nature is blooming, you are feeling part of nature, feeling so comfortable and harmonic. (*give it a moment*)

Notice the beautiful pond, such a wonderful place, walk past it and see that wonderful tree...remembering those wonderful insights...keep walking slowly and almost floating...

162

(If continued from Part 1 start here with desired level of relaxation)

There is a lovely bench close by and you can easily get there and sit down very comfortable feeling free and at peace. Notice someone walking towards you in the distance. It feels good. You might know the person, you might not. It doesn't matter. This person walks towards you and you feel there is something special and kind about this situation. You look forward to this encounter.

Can you describe the person? *(gender, clothes etc.)*

Invite him/her/it to sit next to you.

We now ask if this person has anything to convey to you...any messages or helpful insights and thoughts.
(Sometimes there is a deceased person and a great way to get a lovely closure. Write these down.)

We ask the person to switch places with you because you need to see what they see. One, two, three...and you have now switched places and you can see yourself through this person's kind eyes. *(give it a moment; these are usually very important moments)*

Tell me what you see? *(if not positive, then look closer, beneath everything, to the beauty inside.)*

Now let's switch back....one, two, three...and you are now back in your body with new insights.

Let's ask this person if there are any words of wisdom or helpful words they wish to convey. *(Sometimes there is an amazing educational conversation going on for several minutes.... let it take that time)*

163

When you feel ready, we thank this person and say goodbye for now. We know we can meet again...just as we did now.

When you are ready, let's walk back to the tree, pass the tree and to the pond. Let's check again if anything is written in the sand...what does it say?
Slowly and very harmoniously, take your time to walk back...feeling absolutely wonderful, enjoying your new insights. Walking towards the door, closing it after you. Positive feelings are filling your whole body...you are feeling great and in a moment, when you are ready, come back to here and now, keeping these wonderful feelings.

Chapter 7 Empowerment and Success

Empowering Suggestions

by Sherry M. Hood

This is a direct suggestion script that is written in the form of positive affirmation statements. We often see positive affirmations written as carefully crafted one liners. I have taken it a little further and crafted many sentences and paragraphs under each individual heading.

As you listen to these empowering suggestions, you have the ability to choose the ones that are right and perfect for you. If anything I say does not resonate with you, you can simply let it go, or you may even decide to change the words within your own mind so that they can benefit you.

Balance

You always take the time that you need to coordinate your life. You never let things weigh you down or stand in your way. In seeking balance, you find your center. You are centered and balanced. Your cheerfulness is contagious. People are drawn to you because of your positive attitude. Your heart is cheerful and everyone around you shares in your joy.

You are a fair and honest person. You are consistently honest in all of your dealings. You approach every situation with an open mind and you always consider what it would be like to be on the receiving end of your actions. You are fair and honest in all that you do. You see life through unbiased eyes. You go deep to find meaning in what is truthful and you are never fooled by appearances. Finding truth is meaningful to you. Your insight grows with each day that passes.

You go forth into life with a feeling of sheer joy. You enjoy each day and you always find the gifts in every situation. You believe in miracles and other wonders. You are spontaneous and filled with a wonderful sense of humour.

You accept the differences in all people that are around you. You honour each individual and you treat every person with dignity and respect. You see the beauty in everyone and you are filled with a deeper understanding. You know when to be still. You easily experience the tenderness of your heart and you constantly experience the beauty around you. You are still and centered, knowing that more can be achieved in thoughtful silence then through unconsidered words and deeds. You are calm, relaxed and tranquil in chaotic situations. There is a quietness within you that nothing can disturb. You are at peace with yourself and everyone around you.

You never become weighed down by worldly forces. You are light and easy at all times. You remain calm and centered at all times, and in all situations. You treat others as you would have them treat you, with respect and the utmost consideration. You pride yourself on this.

Caring

You are understanding, patient and you act responsibly towards everyone around you. You always act with great kindness and tenderness. You have many talents which you honour and share with others. You look upon your talents as gifts that you continue to nurture and because of this, they always grow and mature to reach their greatest potential.

You always look at yourself through loving eyes. You are filled with self respect and love for you know that you are steadily moving forward. You are constantly growing and learning. You are part of the global family and you realize this fully and completely. Your heart is open and you accept your part in helping to alleviate the suffering of members of your extended global family. It is your nature to give and you do so unconditionally. You give from your heart. You are generous and kind.

You are clear minded and focused at all times. You are easily able to go within and receive guidance and inspiration as you need it. You look upon each moment as a learning experience. You are always willing to learn and grow. Knowledge gives you clear understanding. You always take responsibility for your own actions. You never overreact.

You see things clearly and you remain calm and centered at all times. You work well with others and you experience the delight of working as a part of a team You are easily able to give and accept help from others.

Harmony

You are in tune and connected with everyone and everything around you. Your purpose is clearly defined and it fills your heart. Your heart is light and full of laughter. You take life in stride. You are careful not to take life too seriously. Your smile is instant and spontaneous. Even your eyes smile. You develop your sense of humour fully now. You are free to be your authentic self.

You allow your own transformation to occur naturally and easily. You realize that you are a constantly growing and maturing person. You never try to transform others. You concentrate on yourself and you will soar. You have great energy, stamina and zeal. Even when you are not thrilled by circumstances, you give your best and you are constantly surprised and amazed by the outcome and the results.

You are always open to new ideas and opinions of others. You are an excellent listener. You encourage others to be open by being open yourself. You are always courteous and sensitive to others around you. You live your life fully and you value every moment of the present. You are straightforward and you always act as yourself. You trust yourself, making it easy to trust others. You can be who you are and allow others that same right.

Health

Your excellent health is improving. Your outlook is improving. You realize that your thoughts control the direction your life takes and you always keep the most positive thoughts for yourself and others.

All systems of your body function naturally and harmoniously. You are a worthwhile and lovable person. You deserve perfect health. You believe in your ability to achieve balanced health. You value your life by living it fully now. You choose to see humour and lightness in your life and you allow this attitude to brighten your life and the lives of those around you.

You realize that your mind is very powerful and there is a mind, body connection. You control your body with your mind and you choose the thoughts that are the best for you.

Today you choose to keep a strong attitude. You are on the road to balanced health and wellbeing. You plunge into life and you get going. Nothing stops you, nothing stands in your way. You absolutely refuse to worry about the future or the past. You always make a difference every day. You continually develop all of the different facets of your life. You are confident and calm in everything that you do.

You have the ability to influence your interactions and thereby you influence the colour of your days. You now resolve problems with direct action. You relax fully in your body and in your mind. You are strong. You now allow yourself the right to change. You can live a healthy, happy life.

You now turn your personal dial to more positive messages. You now develop strong, healthy habits. As you love your body, it in turn works right for you. You are happy and you feel good about yourself. You have the freedom to imagine whatever you want and you realize that what you think determines the direction your life will go in.

You have the ability to set new goals. All things are manageable. Your expectations are realistic and obtainable. Courage opens the door to wisdom and peace of mind. You now consider your wellness. You now choose to give yourself room to grow. You now become confident in your ability to live a good life. You now set yourself free.

Prosperity

You have completely discarded any thoughts of failure that you used to have. You have your goals, aims and objectives well defined and organized. You organize your goals by writing each of them down, along with the steps that you need to make in order to reach them.

You can allow abundance into your life. You can invite abundance into your life. You allow yourself the right to have abundance in your life. You are enthusiastic and positive in everything that you do. You look at every situation as an adventure and you are easily able to see things through a new lens. You seek the deeper meaning in everything around you. You easily flow with change.

You are open to the unlimited possibilities that are there for you. You never limit yourself by the short sighted beliefs of others. You are flexible. You easily discard unnecessary information so that you can move forward towards the essence of each situation. You think through each situation that comes your way. You realize that your actions today will affect your life tomorrow. You always do the very best for yourself, today and into the future.

Wisdom

Knowledge, insight and good judgment are developed when you reflect on the experiences in your life. As you live a life that is filled with meaning and purpose, your wisdom continues to grow and mature. You have the strength and courage to endure difficult times. You always listen to your inner voice. You trust in it and you move forward constantly. You act with dignity and respect in everything that you do. People like being around you because you are self assured and positive.

You are able to view situations at a distance without allowing your emotions to cloud the issue at hand. You are fair and unbiased in all that you do. You have unlimited capabilities. Your self confidence and self esteem grow and mature with each day that passes. You believe in yourself. You are easily able to see issues on a different level. You consider all the facts before you make a decision. You can rest assured that you have made the right choice.

Determination

You never allow anyone or anything stand in your way or keep you from achieving your goals and desires. You are organized and prepared. You know how to prioritize. You are confident in your abilities. You are clear in your objectives and you know your work very well. What you do today will help you tomorrow. You never dwell in the past. You move forward into the future with a clear mind and a plan. Problems are your teachers. You learn from them. You discover what you need to do and when to do it.

You never allow the outside world to influence you in a negative way. Your inner world is peaceful and steadfast, even when the outside is filled with chaos and confusion. You are strong and focused. You are able to deal with anything that comes your way.

Your talents, skills and abilities are like flowers that you have been growing your entire life. You nurture these flowers in order to fulfill your life purpose. You are focused and in complete control. You stay on a clear path. You know what to do, how to do it and when to do it.

Qualities

Your days are filled with joy and happiness. As you put forth positive energy, positive energy returns to you. You are surrounded by positive people, positive places and positive situations. By living happily, you are constantly surrounded by special moments.

You are calm, relaxed and centered, knowing that everything happens in its own time, as it should be. You always enjoy the present moment. You radiate love and happiness. Your entire being is love. You have faith and confidence knowing that you will always make the very best of every situation. You are optimistic and enthusiastic in everything you do. Peace, love and joy surround you at all times.

You move through life in the gentlest way. You calm those you meet along the way with your wonderful, gentle manner. You believe in the everlasting magic of life. You are filled with hope and guided by inspiration, knowing that you are always moving forward.

Success: Creating and Embracing It

by Cynthia da Silva

You are here...right now...because you are ready to take your life to a whole new level. You are ready...to make your mark. You have more potential...and more power...than you ever imagined. You are already on your path of success...because you have already made the move...to take charge...to take control...to create...and embrace...your own...success.

You have dreams. You have goals. You have unique ideas and great imagination. And you are passionate...and driven.

Successful people know...that they can't just sit back...and wait...wait for something to happen...or...wait for the 'right' opportunity to come along.

It's your choice...to either sit back and wait....wait and see what happens TO you. OR...to take action...and MAKE it happen. Instead of...being an observer...of your own life...you can be...the creator.

The choice is yours. The power...is yours. You have the power...to create...the life that you desire...and deserve. Because there is no one in the world...exactly like you, you bring your own unique ideas and abilities to everything you do.

You were born with the incredible and wonderful power...of imagination...which is available to you at all times...to access...and activate...at will. Your own imagination...along with your own personal layers of knowledge and experience...combine to make you...the unique person that you are.

Successful people believe in themselves. They believe...in their abilities and their ideas. They believe in their goals. YOU...believe in yourself...even if others may doubt you.

You believe in your own...unique abilities, ideas and goals.

Successful people have passion....a burning desire. They maintain a feeling of excitement...every day. They stay driven and motivated...until they achieve...whatever it is...they have set their sights on.

You easily find your passion. And you thoroughly feel that passion...every day. Whether it is a well-thought-out goal...or even just a seed of an idea...you generate excitement for it...and you keep that excitement...growing stronger and stronger...every day. You stay passionate, focused...and motivated.

Successful people find it easy to define their goals. They set their sights on their goals...and they stay inspired...and focused on achieving those goals. You easily define and determine your goals. You generate a constant stream of thoughts and ideas. Your life is a continual series of dreams, ideas, goals and accomplishments.

Successful people...are not deterred by obstacles or fear or self-doubt. As you continue along your path to success...there will be obstacles...but you do not mind. You see those obstacles as exciting challenges. You have the ability...to overcome...any obstacle that appears in your path. Your confidence and your abilities...will see to it.

Whenever there are roadblocks or problems...you easily find

solutions...then keep moving forward. Whether the obstacle comes from an outside source or from within...you easily move past it.

Successful people...are not afraid of a challenge. YOU...are not afraid of a challenge...in fact...you welcome it. Each challenge...gives you the opportunity to be creative...to gather inspiration to display...your own wisdom and power. When faced with a challenge...you instinctively know....just what to do.

For any question...you find an answer. For any problem you find a solution. New ideas, answers and solutions...easily flow through you. If you stumble and fall...you get right back up...stronger than ever...even more determined...even more passionate...even more driven.

Along the way...there may be momentary feelings of doubt or fear or insecurity. That is when you will remind yourself...of your amazing confidence and strength. You have no intention of being stopped. You are reminded that you have unlimited potential. You are also reminded...that you are in control...of your own thoughts...at all times. And you can easily push away any negative, fearful or limiting thoughts. You can simply imagine them as a light going out, fading out and fading away. And you automatically replace those undesirable, negative thoughts with positive, empowering, strengthening thoughts.

From time to time ...you may decide that you need to re-evaluate your goals...or to regroup in some way. You instinctively know what adjustments need to be made. You may decide to let go of whatever no longer works...or no longer suits you. At any time...at any moment...you can make a new start...from right where you are. You know that the path of success is never a straight line. There will be twists and turns...but that just makes it all the more exciting. You remain sure of yourself.

Successful people...keep the faith alive. You keep the faith...that what you want is within your reach. Always keeping the faith...you remind yourself...that you are capable...you are worthy...you are deserving. Yes, you believe in yourself and your ideas and goals...even if others seem to doubt you. You trust your own inner guidance and wisdom. You keep that faith in yourself...as you maintain your sense of confidence and power. You consistently stay inspired and driven. You are on your own path of success. Discovering your own potential, you chart your course with conviction. You keep your goals firmly planted in your mind. It is about taking action...and confidently continuing on your path...each day...constantly moving...in the direction...of your goals and dreams. You are here to show the world what you have to offer.

Everything is falling together...even better than you imagined. You embrace your success. You enjoy your success. You are proud of your success. And you are an inspiration to others. Bursting with unlimited potential...you ARE success!

A Script for Procrastination or Chronic Lateness

by Michelle Braun

Utilizes a combination of Contextual Hypnosis and Advanced Neuro Noetic Hypnotherapy techniques, with a touch of Ho'oponopono and some wording that allows for incorporation of EFT as homework if practitioner desires.

Since "parts" of a person are mentioned in script, be sure to fully discuss concept of "parts" prior to induction. (We all have parts of us that want to do or not do something. Give several examples. Make certain client understands this concept completely before beginning hypnosis.)

Following induction:

Deepener 1: Progressive Muscle Relaxation integrating Mindfulness *(wording such as: with each breath, here and now, you notice these things and other useful things, paying attention to sensations, etc...)*

Deepener 2: Staircase

Visualize, picture, imagine or pretend...a very safe...very secure...well...lit staircase of twenty steps...and visualize, imagine or pretend you see yourself standing at the top of that staircase... you feel very calm and safe...with a white safety stripe across the top stair...these twenty steps... go down...one flight...to the next floor...down...as you prepare to walk...down...you notice something behind you...being curious...you turn around...a beautiful mirror...the frame...very intricately painted...you want to examine

177

it...going towards the mirror...looking at the frame...noticing...something...a bit different...about your reflection...when you realize...you are seeing...that old part of you...that is late or procrastinates...unwanted behavior...cast off...which you can...leave behind...at this very moment...decisively turning your back...to the mirror... turning your back...on unwanted things or behaviors...leaving those behind...now...you can begin...moving forward...your journey...down...the stairs...with feelings or habits anew...

Beginning...even as you place your hand on the handrail...here...starting again...noticing...the white stripe across the top step...reminding you of the starting line of races...you cross...to start...going down...the staircase with your left foot at 19...breathing deeply...calmly...and each and every time...18...downward...feeling more deeply relaxed...as you place your hand on the hand railing...17...calmly confident with your...deeper...resolve...or...16...firmly put your foot down...15...going further down...safely down...the stairs...moving further forward...15...deeper and deeper...more comfortably so...14 ... more relaxed...even more fully and deeply resolved...in leaving unwanted habits or behaviors...13...deeper still...far, far behind you...12... moving forward...breathing more and more deeply...fully relaxed...11...going further and further down...more and more confident...10...even deeper...down...you know this is true...9...with each hand or foot...down...more completely relaxed...8...more deeply calm...with full and complete resolve...7...deeper and deeper...knowing this to be true...6...with every hand or foot going down further...5...more deeply...completely calm...3...breathing more and more comfortably...deeper and deeper into relaxation...and peace...0...and going yet further...even deeper...now...so very deeply relaxed...

And as you arrive...here...at the bottom of the stairs...more and more deeply relaxed...with ease...you can go within yourself...to a peaceful place inside...a place of wisdom and comfort...realizing that you have made a very important decision...becoming aware of all reasons...and all possible solutions...maybe even finding it easier to choose to put off procrastination...to a later time and date...

Isn't that right?...Life is often like a race people choose to run...We decide to practice and practice...because people...sooner or later...do experience an enjoyable feeling of picking up momentum and speed...At first, you're slow...but do it more and more...you become faster and faster...finding it increasingly easier and easier...to complete all necessary steps along the way...gaining competence and speed...quicker and quicker still...in time...you arrive at the big day...ready to go...to win...or just...finish on time...and as you run the race...you choose to gain speed...at just the right time...that is right for you...and perhaps you can make a mental note...of this right time...the goals you achieve...projects you complete...appointments easily kept...the time lines you choose to surpass with success...comfort and ease...as you continue to choose to put off that procrastination to a later time and date...and all the while with each breath you take in this moment...note the feelings you have...or the pictures in your mind of these things...or the words you say to yourself or hear...as you write this note in your mind... back now...even more completely relaxed...towards completion and achievement... of goals...projects...appointments...or even of delaying procrastination and lateness...

You choose to wait until you finish first...and as you finish this note now...you decide to put it on your forehead...and each and every time you look into a mirror...from this time forward...more and more...each and every day you note...you can imagine seeing these things very well a...head...seeing the part of you that schedules yourself with plenty of advance note...ice(*notice*)...and feeling your selected...completely successful end point...as you arrive on time...allowing yourself to later put off putting off even sooner...you don't have to learn how to use these skills...to feel confident...that you complete your race...you just are...as you run down the clock in 10, 9, deeper into time and space of your mind...8, 7, closer and closer to your chosen arrival point at destination...6, 5...of successfully ever deep relaxation...4, 3...more and more...deeply relaxed, calm and confident...2, 1 ... as you approach the beginning of the...0...end...

That's right...completely and deeply relaxed...more than ever before...as you see, hear and feel the joy of completion...double the exhilaration of the end...and achievement of the forward ultimate end goal...as you choose to **jump** onto the finish line...of the deciding race...just in time...or earlier....you win...**noting**...the big smile on your face...from satisfaction you feel as you shout to yourself...now...I DID IT!!...Hear the congratulations you...and others...give yourself...for a race well run, didn't you?...I wonder if you can tell the difference now...or...next time you admire...your own strengths as you reach the finish line on time or before...from all your practice and competency that you chose to create...from all resources that you really knew you had inside...waiting to speed you along...to run your chosen race...but don't finish too soon...

You choose to complete so much more...so easily early all the while...you feel so much more at ease and comfortable...as you decide to arrive with time to spare...when...maybe you can remember, or even remember to forget...how to be late or putting things off to the last moment...and you know...more and more...each and every time you begin preparing your self... you can tap tap tap into this feeling of complete accomplishment...as you breathe...just like your feet tap tap tap as you run the race...you tap into inner success with each and every breath you take...you notice decidedly increasing ease and confidence...with each finger you tap...as you move well along...you breathe...and decide to be on time sooner even now...and feel you can tap into your readiness to begin...a new race in life...each time...imagine yourself...readily deciding...accepting deadlines...as your finish lines for easy success...to be on time sooner even now...with each pen or pencil...you tap or touch in thought...you easily choose...to see the finish line...even more easily approachable...

With each coming breath...each event...deciding...arriving in this time...makes this more and more real to you...as you hear your approach towards...as if your feet are hitting the ground...picking up more and more speed and momentum...and the quicker you go...the more and more easily this becomes your selected lifestyle...this feeling of winning...your personal race is liberating... and perhaps you even notice...that you are able to...choose quickly...easily...successfully...deciding to flick off...putting off...just like flicking off...beads of sweat as you run your race...you can complete so much more...making excellent time moving forward...to continue on to cross the finish line...as you choose to continue to put...off putting...off...

Until you **jump** onto the finish line once again...on

time...and tap it with your hand...you realize your other hand...has already crossed...met your goal...earlier first...because sometime soon...in just the right time... now...you again notice...looking a...head...observing a tri-fold mirror...just a...head...like the old-fashioned vanity mirrors...noticing three images of yourself...perhaps even noticing the old you in the center again...that part having made you miss so much...while the well-trained, practiced and confident you that competently wins...any timed event on either the left or right side...your choice...and the current you...the one that is becoming...that is listening to my words now...on the other side remaining...

Soon I will count upwards, bringing you back to the here and now...but first...it is time now to close the face of this matter...looking a...head...Take the here and now you on that chosen side of the mirror...and fold that here and now part over...and into the center that old was behind...saying as you do this...I love you...I'm sorry...please forgive me...thank you...and maybe you even notice...feeling, hearing and seeing...that old part is happily much further behind you...at...this...very...moment...now...congratulating you for all races done here and...now...or in the future as...you run and win or finish right on time...because it is so very easy to pace yourself at the now and a...head...maybe even joining in to finish...your choices in deciding...just...on...time... here...Making the next fold...of the mirror...where all parts of you...come well placed...on time...together again...and by placing the well practiced...confident you...winner of all timed events...the smooth...easy, confident...calmly self-paced...you in the forefront...on top...you can see a...head all finish lines...making good time now and always... even then you note it is as easy as...changing from your slippers or dress shoes or...work shoes...into your walking or running shoes...because this is an important choice... really...between you...and your own inner self...isn't it?

Notable Networker

by Sue Bridgman

A script designed to improve a person's ability to feel comfortable and confident making new business contacts.

Taking 5 deep breaths, begin with breath one, breathing deeply....hold it...and now exhale...you are becoming deeply relaxed. Take your second deep breath...hold it...and exhale...do this three more times, breathe deeply...hold it...and exhale...When you feel comfortable...give yourself permission to close your eyes...enjoy focusing on the relaxed feeling with each and every breath you take, and as you exhale, breathe out and let go of any tension, problems, or worries of the day...

When you finish taking your fifth breath...focus your attention to the heaviness of your shoes...Even your socks start to feel heavy on your feet...Your shoes and socks, not being normal to your regular body weight...feel very foreign and heavy...This heavy relaxation, starting from your toes and moving up to your heels and ankles will start to become very noticeable...This prominent feeling of heaviness is moving upward into the calves of your legs...your legs, feeling very heavy, are pushing down. This pushing down feeling causes your legs to become deeply relaxed...This relaxed feeling moves to your knees, flowing up into your thighs and hips and throughout your torso. As you focus your concentration on this heavy relaxation, you hear only my voice.

Pay no attention to the sounds inside or outside the room...except for the sound of my voice...for these sounds are simply every day sounds of life...They cannot sidetrack or disturb you, but rather, these noises allow you to fall even deeper into heavy relaxation...

Feel your stomach muscles relaxing...deeply relaxing...your chest area is soaking in relaxation...As you sit deeply relaxed...you notice how your breathing becomes gentle... rhythmic...and you begin to drift into the drowsy... sleepy...daydreaming feeling of relaxation...You allow yourself to give into this feeling and let go of any tensions of the day...and begin to think about how wonderful and amazing you can feel...that drowsy relaxed feeling allows you to go deeper and deeper...and your arms, hands and fingers are feeling a numb...pleasant...tingling feeling.

It is such a pleasant feeling that you find yourself slipping deeper into this relaxation...It spreads to your neck and your forehead...All of the muscles are letting go...Even the tiny muscles in your eyelids...and down to your jaw muscles...are relaxing deeply and growing heavier.

In a moment, I am going to count from 5 – 0 and as I count down, I want you to imagine taking an enjoyable walk on a path. Allow yourself to see all the details in your mind. Using all your senses to hear the sounds, see the colors and your surroundings, smell the smells. When I reach 0, allow yourself to step into this amazing experience while allowing your body to feel deeply relaxed and comfortable.

5 – doubling your relaxation with every step you take on the path
4 – with each breath sinking you further into relaxation, noticing the smell of the fresh clean air, the brightness and clarity of the nature around you.
3 - you are feeling so comfortable and at ease. The beauty of your surroundings cause you to smile with gratitude.
2 – feeling even better as you take in your surroundings and start to feel a bountiful feeling of joy, calmness, and serenity.

1 – focus your attention to how calm...confident...and relaxed you are...as the path leads you up a hill and ends at a manicured lawn where groups of people are socializing.
0 – deep relaxation...
Now...let your thoughts focus upon your desire to connect with people...upon your desire to feel confident around all people...because you are in control. You are in control of how you speak, your gestures, what you say and how you say it. You are in complete control of the way you connect with people.

You are feeling confident and empowered...each step towards the people brings you a sense of satisfaction of the productiveness that is about to take place...You are that much closer to the reason you are on this journey.

And you notice that if any nervousness enters your mind or body, you automatically and effortlessly breathe it away, pressing your index finger and your thumb together to join your calming breath in releasing the stress...quickly and naturally...because you are in control.

You hear the laughter, and see the smiles as a group of people are greeting each other with handshakes...With a smile on your face...you approach the group. You are confident and empowered in every way...Your heart is focused on adding value to others with what you do...As you extend your hand and greet the members in the group, you intentionally focus on listening to each person...making mental notes of their name, business, and aspects of their business...

You are genuinely curious about these people and their business...and it shows as you are actively listening. Your passion for connecting with the people shines through...

After a couple hours of successful networking, you have gathered a lot of cards, names, and gained new relationships...feeling grateful...empowered...and energized... you are now ready to head home. As you head back to the path, you feel energized...refreshed...and renewed. You are excited to follow up with these people and form new and mutually rewarding relationships.

From this day forward, you will no longer be intimated by the crowds...the conversations...and the idea of networking...because you know it is important to you and your business and you have all the resources and control within you.

Each and every day going forward...every time you think you are feeling anxious about or before a networking event...simply press together your index finger and your thumb...and you will feel a calmness and confidence flow over your mind and body...putting you in a wonderful state of ease.

You have done a fantastic job, learning new skills and creating a state of intuition...creativity...and confidence...It is now time to reorient to the room around you...Although your eyes remain shut for a moment...sense the chair below you...and feel the floor below your feet...As you become more aware of the room around you...continue to appreciate the state of hypnosis you created. As I count from 0 to 5...with each number...allow yourself to become aware of the room around you.....feeling more refreshed...with a positive sense of well-being...

0 – Let's close that door to the subconscious mind to block all negatives
1 – slowly and calmly coming up out of the state of hypnosis
2 – physically aware and mentally alert
3 – coming up even higher now
4 – eyes beginning to open and
5 – Eyes Open and Wide Awake, feeling refreshed and renewed

Brilliant Performance

by Patricia Eslava Vessey

Whether you are an athlete, artist or other type of performer, regular participation in this hypnosis process will help you perform, brilliantly, confidently and consistently.

Induction:

Take a deep breath in, and as you let it go...close your eyes down...and before you allow yourself to go into a comfortable trance now, you may want to think about what that means to you...As you allow your entire body to soften and relax...every bone, every tendon, every ligament, every cell in your body softened and relaxed... and with your next deep breath, you can just let those eyes relax so deeply and so comfortably that they just want to remain closed and relaxed, even though you know you could open them if you wanted to, but you just can't be bothered to even try...as they become heavier and heavier with relaxation...

And you can let yourself release any tension or discomfort in your body...while another part of you discovers how wonderful it is to be more relaxed and comfortable now...

And as you rest there, you might wonder if both arms will grow heavier...or lighter...or one arm will grow heavier while the other grows lighter...or perhaps one hand will become warmer or cooler...and you fully give yourself permission to go into a deep trance at your own pace...now...as you relax even more...

And you might be amazed at how easily you drift into a deeper level of trance...And I wonder if you will simply allow it to occur...or your unconscious mind will create a deeper state of comfort...or perhaps you will go deeper and deeper into trance without even knowing how...you are doing it...now...

And you don't even have to notice how supported your body feels as you gently relax every bone, every muscle, every tendon, every fiber...every cell in your body softened and relaxed...While everything begins to just slow down...slow down and relax...and the more you relax, the more you can relax...just allowing and noticing everything slow down...and I wonder if you are noticing just how deeply you are relaxing... how your breathing has changed...how it has slowed down...as you continue to relax more and more...

And you might wonder what it would be like to continue to an even deeper level of trance...feeling so peaceful and relaxed...From the top of your head all the way to the tips of your toes you are relaxed and at ease...And maybe you can notice how wonderful you feel...Allowing even your mind to slow down now...

And as I count from 10 down to 1, I'd like you to go 100 times deeper, quickly, at your own pace, with each number I count...

10 relax...relax...feeling better and better about everything in your life the more relaxed you become...**9** deeper...the more relaxed you get, the better you feel, the better you feel, the more confident and at peace you become...**8** down deeper...becoming more and more clear about why you are here and what you are here to do...and how it becomes more and more important with every day that passes...**7** you have a purpose...you know this at some level and it is becoming clearer and clearer as you drift deeper and deeper...**6** the more relaxed you become, the more aware you become of why you wake up every day...down, deeper and deeper...**5** and it may come to you quickly or within the next few days...down, deeper...**4** down and down, but when you're aware you will know why, what and how...and you will know exactly what you need to do as your motivation increases...**3** down deeper and deeper with ease, drifting and drowsy, drowsy and drifting...**2** down deeper, relaxed...**1** down, down, down, deeper and deeper into total and complete relaxation as you continue to relax...

Suggestions:

Now that you are relaxed and at ease your mind is open to the suggestions I'm about to give you, because this is what you want, these are your goals, to be the person you want to be...to be a brilliant performer...

Now I'd like you to see, sense or imagine a person who has the performance abilities you desire... someone who's performance you want to imitate...someone you, perhaps, admire...bring that person to mind...imagine them now performing - right there in front of you... (*pause*)

Now I want you move closer and study them...watch how they move....notice their gestures...how they are standing... how they use their arms, legs, head...notice how they are using their body as they perform...see those abilities you desire... imagine what's going through their mind...what they might be saying inside as they are performing...and as you are studying that performer, perhaps you can even sense how they are breathing...take it all in - getting a sense and a flow of the rhythm and the sights and sounds of the performance...

As you study that performer, get a sense of those skills, techniques and abilities you would like to possess at the same or even greater skill level...

Now walk around behind the performer, and step fully into their body...that's right, imagine becoming one with that performer...imagine performing and seeing through the eyes of brilliance...feeling that brilliance...moving in their body, your body...feeling their performance...arms, legs, head, entire body...saying those words inside as you are performing in that brilliant way with those abilities...feel what it's like to be performing, confidently, brilliantly, consistently, just the way you want...and as you are doing this your unconscious mind is now learning...integrating...all that you are experiencing and learning and updating your neurology with new skills and abilities...and a knowing that you are now choosing to use these new abilities consistently, confidently, brilliantly each and every time you perform...

And as you step outside that performer's body, you retain all the learning, memories and experiences of performing brilliantly...

Now, imagine your next performance, and as you do, step fully into that performance with all that you have learned from the brilliant performer...see, sense and imagine yourself performing with those abilities becoming stronger...

Now recall a time when you performed brilliantly...another time in your life...think about that event, and remember how you felt...step into those feelings now and, then double those wonderful feelings...turn those feelings up....and then remember what was going through your mind as you performed brilliantly...what did you say to yourself as you were feeling so good...repeat those words now and say even more positive words to yourself as you are reliving this event and feel your confidence, passion and excitement increase...

You are now tapping into a greater level of potential, and it is getting easier and more enjoyable to perform...every practice session your focus becomes more finely tuned...your internal dialogue more confident and certainty occupies each and every cell in your body...your energy level is increasing every day, even right now as you hear my voice you are feeling excited about performing...your physical body will communicate with your mental body in the perfect way necessary for brilliant performance...

When you sleep your body will heal, renew, repair and energize you for your next brilliant performance...every day your desire for healthy food, proper hydration, exercise and other healthy habits is getting stronger leading you to make more and more healthy choices...your thirst for success in performing brilliantly is increasing every day...

After every practice and performance you communicate more effectively and supportively with yourself to make any adjustments necessary in order to maintain a greater degree of balance, both physically and emotionally as your performance continues to improve...

Imagine sitting down to watch your performance event on TV...As the performance begins, you realize that you are the one performing...see yourself performing brilliantly...and perhaps you can even feel it in your body, realize the confidence and see the pride that is now yours with each and every performance...

All these suggestions are becoming a permanent part of your inner reality, impacting your performance in ways you desire...for good...you now will stay focused and centered as you perform...you are experiencing a greater degree of control over your entire body...you are making all necessary corrections automatically for optimum performance leading to a brilliant performance every time you perform.... Know that you are here for a reason...you are capable of great things and you are easily, passionately, confidently stepping into that role now...

Now, it is almost time to return to full awareness. Each and every suggestion that you accept now becomes a permanent part of your unconscious mind. They become a part of your thoughts, your behavior, and your being....part of your personality. Each time you participate in this process you enter this state of relaxation quickly, easily and effortlessly. Accepting everything that is positive and beneficial for you and releasing anything that does not fit into your life at this time.

Reaching Your Potential through Creative Ideas

by Linda Roan

Ask client beforehand if are they comfortable with animals...Following induction of your choice:

Stepping onto the garden porch now of an old, old house...knowing you are entering a tranquil, peaceful place...let your senses guide you...your sense of taste, your sense of smell...your sense of touch...of sight...all enhancing your wonderful imagination...now imagine yourself sitting in a large, comfortable chair of the porch...breathing in and out easily, comfortably...

Surrounding you on the floor of the porch are clay pots...filled with the crimson blossoms of geraniums...and the trailing scent of honeysuckle knotted with garlands of butter coloured flowers...the light green flavours and scents of herbs mingle in a moss encrusted herb planters...

Before you stretches a beautiful garden...full of rose bushes heavy with ripe, deep pink and white blooms, strong oaks shelter posies of mottle faced pansies and frilly skirted marigolds...nearby surf blue irises...gilded by the sun, nod and gather in a dancing circle of reeds around a small pond...

It has been a warm, summer's day which is slowly coming to a close as the sunlight begins to fade. The colours of the trees and plants around you are beginning to soften in the fading light.

Everything is quiet except for the bees peacefully buzzing

around the small petals of the fragrant lavender bushes...and the sound of the gentle breathing of a favourite pet...real or imagined lying by your side...reach down and feel with your hand the light rise and fall of your pet's breath through its comforting body...

In the distance, on a sturdy oak tree the bird feeder lazily sways as the last few sparrows gather...their only sound their russet tipped feathers flickering faintly as they feed.

At your side is a small table covered with a beautiful lace cloth...on the table is a bowl of glistening, ripe fruit. Reach towards the bowl and pick up your favourite piece of fruit...bite into the fruit and enjoy its sweet, juicy flavour.

All around you the air is warm and soothing. The blue grey sky of the closing evening is threaded with lingering sun rays...listen to the low, soft rustle of a breeze through the leaves. As the petals of the roses begin to close for the night, watch some of them drift on to the small pond, sprinkling the water and its lilies with a confetti of pink and white...drifting, drifting...this way and that, that way and this...all the way down, down, down...further and further...

Now imagine those small petals represent the wonderful, creative...intuitive ideas and solutions floating around in the deep, rich earth of your fertile subconscious...and that the following beneficial suggestions I am about to give you are going to sink deeply into this deep rich earth...causing them to begin working immediately and powerfully and these suggestions become more effective each day...

Continuing to relax even more deeply...knowing the deeper levels of your subconscious mind and your connection to the collective subconscious, the universal mind contains all the knowledge, talents and skills which you have gathered and developed as a result of your years of experience...from the time you came into existence...you have been soaking up countless impressions...and forming beliefs about yourself and others...bringing with you the ancestral memories in your dna...creating positive memories and ideas...and you now have a great deal of insight and experience...as well as your inner wisdom...

And all of that knowledge, all of those talents and gifts are in every level of your subconscious mind and in your connection to the collective subconscious, the universal mind and all that information is available to be used by you creatively and intuitively...achieving your full potential...

Sports Performance - Hockey

by Sheila Wardman

Here are two versions of hockey performance enhancement. The second is specific for the goalie.

As you go deeper, I would like you to see yourself in your favorite hockey game...you are not particularly interested...at this specific moment...in achievement or in failing. But rather...just being fully involved in the game you enjoy. Let yourself...just be fully immersed in this adventure...put on the skates, the gear, the gloves, the pads...put on whatever things there are that go with hockey...Just be for a moment...fully dressed...in the gear for hockey...all that this game requires...

Feel yourself there, totally prepared ready for the game you are about to play. Now, I would like you to visualize in your mind, as clearly as you can... it will become clearer for you as you go deeper....you're going deeper now. See yourself in the middle of the hockey game that you love so much...I want you to go deeper and go deeper...Letting yourself, allowing yourself to get more in touch with how it feels to be in the game...how your body feels to be in this game. Until the game becomes so real for you, that it's as if you are in the middle of the best hockey game ever...it could be the Olympics...just put yourself there now.

It's unavoidable now, for you not to be in the middle of it...and you don't want to avoid it...you just give permission to yourself...to be fully in the moment. Experiencing the scents...the sounds...the emotions...the feelings...the joy...the exhilaration of what that feels like to be there...now.

Being fully in this game, you notice some things that not everybody has noticed. And, in fact, you may not have noticed them yourself before. You notice...that there are particular times in this sport where you seem to have boundless energy. You seem to be able to move so smoothly and so effectively...your skating strides are very intentional...each one propels you faster and faster to get to that puck.

I want you to pay particular attention to those moments...they are special moments...and I want you to notice something else as well...that all you need to do now is to focus on these moments...of grace...heightened awareness...of pucks going into the opposing net...of scoring many goals that seem so effortless, so easy....players from the opposing team skate to you...you know where they are...your senses are finely tuned to them approaching...You bump them off the puck or into the boards...You are at ease...you know you have this innate inner sense of everything going on around you. You notice the skill at which you can handle everything in these moments...effortlessly and easily.

Your skating strides are smooth and powerful...you turn quickly when you need to...stopping is instantaneous. Any change of direction has a flow to it. Such skill is available to you anytime. Your backward skating is powerful and fluid. It's available from the very fiber of your being, and it is not difficult for you to find this. You may also notice that you're not quite up to par. You will notice there is still room for you to improve your abilities here. You notice that sometimes there will be things on your mind that will distract you.

There may be times when you'll become fearful and apprehensive that others are beating you to the puck or you are avoiding being hit, or will say things that are not positive, or maybe the competition will overtake you, or overcome you, and for that reason these energies are circumvented.

But you notice something...now that you have available to you that you've never had before...and that is an ability to turn off, just like one turns the handle of a water faucet off...all fear, all worry and all self-doubt. I want you to see the tap being opened and any fear...anxiety...failure and competition running out that spout, pouring itself onto the ground, making a huge puddle of water. I want you to reach over with all of your strength and all of your ability and turn the faucet off. And as you turn that faucet off...I want you to notice the strength you have.

It is not as if there is nothing ever to worry about, it's just that you decide this is not the time to be worrying. And you decide that worrying does not change the way in which you play the game. And so, as you decide this, and you notice there is no more water, no more fear, there is nothing else draining away your energy...the sun comes out and the water dries up.

Until moments ago, it may have seemed like a flood, but now all before you is clear, is dry...perfectly available for you. You notice in this experience that you can turn off all that interferes with your well-being in the middle of your game. You can also turn ON the energy of the natural sun that is within you....that source that has the light to power each and every muscle completely and perfectly.

In the future...when you are preparing yourself for the

game...readying yourself...to be completely present in the moment...that you so much enjoy and are so connected to...you spend a moment with your eyes closed and say to yourself,

"I allow the sunrise of my own strength, the sunrise of my own energy, the sunrise of my own victory to come up and to totally, completely dry up all the fear and all the doubt. To take away all the hesitation of this sport of hockey, and to lead me clearly, quickly and smoothly to full and complete enjoyment, involvement and positive action."

You know now that you can excel at hockey and to do so is effortless and easy. You move forward without doubt and without fear. And every day that you practice this exercise and you do practice, you want to practice, you love it...you notice allowing the sunrise of your own strength, allowing the light to illuminate who it is you really are...you allow yourself to have more positive and wonderful experiences...

Your body becomes finely tuned; every muscle works exactly as you would like it to work. All the cells in your body are energized to the frequency and intentions you send to them...all positive, in unison with the feel of working together on the greatest game in history. And you recognize the level of mastery that is yours...you embrace mastery, being the best you can be, having a sense and a feeling that you do everything to support the team you are playing with...your passing of the puck is fluid and stick to stick...your team mates are congratulating you for the great plays you are making.

You are winning in the greatest game ever! Your confidence soars like an eagle just floating on the wind. You are so there...in the game. Loving it...you truly... completely...enjoy it.

Here is a script for helping a goalie enhance performance:

As a goalie, I focus on the puck and play at all times. I visualize or imagine myself goaltending in the greatest Hockey game ever. It could be the Olympics. I put myself there now...in the Olympics, imagining or visualizing...the sights...the sounds...the smells...the people...the energy. I soak in the energy...

The puck drops... I turn my head to follow the puck...I continue following the puck...as it bounces...I quickly and easily recover the rebound. I create the habit of turning my head and watching every puck that is hit...I react quickly and easily...I realize that tracking the puck...allows me...the ease of stopping it!

I see how easily this gives me a jump on stopping the rebound. I recover the puck...making a great save. Making the first save is easy. I control the rebound...I always recover the puck. I have a heightened sense of awareness...in a game...I make the save. I instinctively react to where the puck bounces...and STOP it...I have a goalie's instinct...I am present to this instinct in practice and in games; I feel it within me...I always practice and play at 100%...I expect to be excellent in any game.

Goalies go after all rebounds...I play intensely...actively...I'm up and I'm down as fast as possible...I have lightening speed. At anytime, another player may be getting ready to shoot. I have plenty of time to see the puck hit...I recover it. I cut off many angles...All this is possible for me. I start with my skates on the middle of the goal line...and as the puck comes over the center line...I turn my chest to face the puck and the shooter...I push to the top of the crease. Now...I have my angle...and I'm ready for the shot...If a pass comes...I'm ready and quick to push to a new angle.

Thinking is for practice...and with our hockey coach...Out on the ice...it's time to let instinct take over...Stay focused. Stay present...I burn a hole in the puck with my laser-focused eyes. I have a laser focus on the puck at all times. At times...I may find my mind wandering a little...I go for a quick skate...to the corners...in between play...with my eyes on the ice...nothing distracts me. I keep aware...of where I need to be...when the puck drops.

I am stopping shots...My play is amazing...I am active and fluid like the best of the NHL goalies. One day I may be an NHL goalie... I practice and play like one. I feel like Carey Price. I imagine myself to take on the abilities of Carey Price. I am excited, present, calm and so tuned in to my game.

I have the perfect mental framework...and focus...I am a great goaltender. It is an honor to play this position...With this honor comes a great deal of responsibility. As a goaltender...I take responsibility for my practice and game preparation...At practice...I am a goaltender that loves the opportunity to work hard...Hard work in practice...leads to a well-prepared goaltender...well-prepared both physically and mentally. A well-prepared goaltender...is a confident goaltender. The harder I work in practice and in games...the more prepared I become.

I am confident. I love this game. My technique is an instinct...it comes to me easily and effortlessly...I can call on my instinct whenever I need to. I am confident in myself...I have strong glove hands...amazing vision...I love this game. I am relaxed...focused...and ready to face all game situations...

I focus with simplicity. I am in a position to be successful every time...Great saves occur...when I allow my natural instincts...and ability to shine. I allow my instincts to shine...they are a gift I possess within me.

As I focus on the next shot...I am in the moment. Next shot...focus...in the moment...focused on what is in my control. Everything is in my control. I own the crease. I communicate with my team. I challenge the shooters. I allow no rebounds. I am a competitor. I keep my intensity. I am playing this position proudly...with a smile inside my heart. I am a winner. This is the greatest position ever...I love being a goaltender. I love this Game.

I am – It is

by June Austin

This is a handout I give out at a Self-Hypnosis or Goal Setting/Dream Achievement Workshop as examples of affirmative "self-programming" for the student's scripting lesson to tailor their own daily self- hypnosis program. I have adapted all of these into sessions with clients...

I am confident, strong and efficient. Each morning I awaken refreshed and energized, I love life.

The more I smile, the better I feel. The better I feel, the easier it is to accomplish my goals. My mind, body and emotions are healthy, strong and balanced.

I have talents and gifts that can benefit others. It is easy to see where I can use them best.

More and more, with each passing day, I can feel my inner worth growing and emerging joyfully in each endeavor (or encounter with someone or something new).

I deserve the best that life has to offer and easily achieve each separate goal as a step toward fulfillment in life. My goals are clear and my thoughts and actions are in complete harmony with them.

I immediately recognize when "old programming" attempts to block my progress. It is easy to decide whether this is a false belief or a true intuitive red flag.

I handle each moment and situation calmly, patiently,

gracefully and diplomatically.

Should I encounter a setback on my journey toward fulfillment, it is clearly an opportunity to sharpen my skills of perseverance and optimism; it provides me with information on how to get to the next step in my life's journey.

The more chaotic situations appear, the more organized, composed and focused I become.

I happily achieve success in everything I plan to do and act on my plans confidently. I appreciatively accept all the warmth, joy and abundance (prosperity) life has to offer. I give thanks for these gifts with thoughts and actions of kindness and generosity.

I stand tall, breathe deeply, smile brilliantly and live each moment to its fullest. I am worthy. I believe in my ability to create and shape my world in harmony with my goals while benefiting others (my loved ones, the planet, my community).

Remember, your subconscious will move you toward what you fill it with: Make your statements in present tense like you are moving toward your goals or already achieving your goals such as "I enjoy city driving. Every trip is pleasant and safe." "Every month, I find I have more and more surplus income. It is easy to meet my obligations and invest this surplus in my goals and dreams."

PLEASE AVOID: Contracted words such as: can't, don't, won't, etc...or use unwanted situations or emotional descriptors such as: "I won't get angry in traffic anymore." or "I am no longer frustrated when I pay my debts."

Chapter 8 Anxiety, Fear and Depression

Fear of Water

by Michelle Braun

The following script is written using the principles of Advanced Neuro-Noetic Hypnosis™. ANNH™ was created and is taught by Tim Brunson of the International Hypnosis Research Institute. According to Brunson, "Advanced Neuro-Noetic Hypnosis™ (ANNH) is the integral mind/body art and science which studies human potential and transformation, combining the latest concepts with neurodynamics, quantum theory, and ancient wisdom."

The short phrase format of this script utilizes the brain's method of pattern recognition and its need to create meaning from the ambiguity created by the looping of suggestions.

How to read this script:

The capitalization at the end of each short phrase replaces punctuation. Each capitalization indicates a pause after the phrase is stated as it is a stand alone thought or suggestion. While each capital letter indicates a break in speech, a practitioner can read it in any manner that is comfortable for them. However, adding more breaks or pauses between some words for emphasis, rather than fewer pauses/breaks, is preferable in this style, but these are not necessarily long pauses. The idea is to read this script as poetry, not prose.

This script is not to be used for phobias. Ensure adequate deepeners are used.

In this very moment You can Listen Or feel your heartbeat You are fine Knowing You are Ready for change Now Old Unused items Trends Or habits Can change overnight Carefully selecting The ones to toss Imagine Being free Make room For wonderful New feelings And memories Maybe notice Heart slower Confident Out with the old In with new Relaxed breathing Comfortable At all times As you remove even more Unwanted things Time to forget to remember Unneeded Useless to you Lost their appeal Relaxing even more Realizing Some nice sweet water helps You decide Life Cannot exist without sun or water Here Now Confidence fills all aspects of life Feeling natural Free Childlike Floating Playing Splashing Because All possibilities exist When you free yourself Make room You can Anything Just Choose A musty Old useless coat Perhaps recalling it Caressing your body Before So easy to feel it there Now As you realize Its time has passed Life can be different Ready for all New things to come Water Comfortably rolls off your body Like bags of useless unwanted items roll into a bin As natural as water runs off a duck You can Choose Be relaxed Comfortable Easily moving through life Or water Necessary for life Be your greatest self As many sweet smiles And warm wanted Hugs from loved ones Shower over you Filling your days Raining success It's only natural Your brain is 80% water Observing you can cool or warm your hands and feet At will More comfortable Relaxed At all times Or when needed Most people Nearly 60% water Happy in Or near Water Comfortable Relaxed Joyful Secure Slowing your breathing breath by breath Perhaps noticing You can Slow it even more As you More happy Joyful In water New life begins in water Yours Naturally too Notice your heartbeat Comfortable Slow Relaxed At ease Secure In the water As comfortable Now Or later Just let it be so Bringing back with you All the new Needed Wonderful Relaxed Happy feelings And all new Wanted memories You've been creating Attain joy It's yours to be had Now and all ways Always It Is Here And now Allow yourself to slowly begin the journey In time right for you Back to the present moment Feeling energized Healthy Calm Well-rested Ready to accomplish When You are ready Open your eyes

Meeting the Anxious Part

by Zoilita Grant

Close your eyes. Take a moment to settle in ... to feel yourself supported... to know that you are in safe place. It's okay to let go. Take in a long, deep breath and hold it...now let it out with a sigh. Take in another long, deep breath ... feeling your chest gently rise as you inhale ...and letting out your breath slowly in your own time and space. Gently close your eyes. (*pause*)

Now I'm going to lead you through a progressive relaxation exercise, which will take you into a deeply relaxed state. I'm going to count backwards from ten to one. Each descending number will take you to a deeper level of your own mind.

10...9...8...go deeper 7...6...5...deeper still...4...3...2...1...you are there!

Now imagine a soft, warm shower of light pouring delightfully over your body, washing away all tension, washing away all pressure. Concentrate your attention upon your scalp, as the tightness dissolves and melts away, allow your scalp to relax completely.

Move the attention slowly downward, focus upon the forehead...feel all the tension drain away as the warm, soothing shower of light washes over your body. The shower creates a tingling, vibrating sensation as it flows gently down your face. (*pause*) Relax your cheeks...relax and let go...relax the jaw...allowing your jaw to gently drop...relaxing and letting go of all your tension.

Feel your ears relax...your eyes...your eyebrows and forehead... feel all the muscles relax and let go. Feel your eyelids relaxing...relaxing and letting go. Breathe deeply and naturally...feeling all the muscles and tissues around your eyes relax. Even the eyeballs themselves are relaxed and letting go. Feel the tension drain down your neck...your shoulders...just release and let go of all the tension and stress...feeling a tingling, vibrating sensation as you let go completely.

Feel the tingling and vibrating sensation in the arms and the hands as you relax them completely. Now let the warm wave flow down the back, drawing with it all the tightness...all the tension.

Take in a nice deep breath, feeling your chest rise gently as you inhale...then relaxing as you exhale. Feel the tingling and vibrating sensations as you exhale. Feel the tension drain away from the neck and shoulder muscles. Release all your tension as you breathe deeply and naturally...Relax the pelvis and the hips, releasing the tension and pressure. Relax all the internal organs, every gland, every cell, and every organ, is functioning in a rhythmic and healthy manner as you release all excess tension and pressure...Let go... Let go...

The soft caressing light is pouring delightfully over your body as you relax the thighs ... the calves...the knees...the feet. Your entire body is completely and totally relaxed. The flowing, soothing light causes a tingling and vibrating sensation to envelope the entire body. Feel your body getting lighter and lighter. Feel as if your body is floating gently ... softy, safely, in a warm, buoyant sea of light...becoming lighter...and lighter...and lighter...(*long pause*)

Feel the warmth and comfort of being safe. You are safe; secure and strong, it is okay to let go. Release the limbs...let them float within the light...the arms and legs feel as if they do not belong to you...the entire body is released and free.

You are comfortable, you are supported...you are safe... you are completely and totally relaxed. (*long pause*)

Now go into your mind and quiet your mind...And it's good to know that you have a conscious and a subconscious... and that is good to know... and it is good to know that the conscious mind can drift now...rest now...drift and rest now.

The subconscious hears and understands everything that I am saying...and I am talking to the subconscious. The subconscious knows how deep you need to be to get maximum benefit from this process today. I now direct the sub-conscious to take you to the right level now!

10...9...8...7...6...5...4...3...2...1 You are there!

Today we are going to go on a journey...a journey to meet (customize to the anxious characteristics of the client) the anxious part of you...That part of you that is vulnerable and needs healing...anxious one...You are standing on a path, a path that leads to a door...the door to the room of the anxious one...there are ten steps to the door...ten steps to the room....the room of the each step takes you closer...closer to the anxious one ...starting to walk to the door now...10-9-8-7-6-5-4-3-2-2-1...standing in front of the door now...the door to the room of the anxious one...on the door it says...Room of the anxious one...it is easy to talk now...

Can you imagine this door? (*wait for client to answer*)

You are your adult self on a very good day, a very strong day and you are connected to your own Spiritual Resources...Are you ready to go into the room? (*wait for the client to answer*)

Go into the room. Can you see or sense or feel (*customize to the client's anxious characteristics*)...the anxious one? (*wait for the client to answer*)

Tell me about the anxious one...Can he/she see you? How does the anxious one feel about you? Ask the anxious one...(*wait for client to answer*)

Come as close to the anxious one as you can ....can you touch her/him? Ask the anxious one what he/she wants to tell you. Listen inside...listen inside...What does the anxious one need/want to say...(*wait for the client to answer...allow time for silent processing*)

(*Create a connection between the anxious one and the adult*) Go deeper now (*give at least one positive suggestions and visualizations designed to help the client feel calm and centered*) Now let's do a mental rehearsal of you in your outer world,. feeling all this calm and centeredness coming from within..supporting and nurturing the anxious one ...it is easy to talk now...can you tell me what that would be like?(*wait for client to answer*)...(*long pause*)

Now, let's take a moment to integrate this process fully into your being...Body, Mind, Spirit and Emotions...and now...integrate...integrate...integrate this connection to the anxious one into the fiber of your being...You are calm, peaceful and centered..

Getting ready to come back now, awake and aware. I am counting to five and when I say five you will be awake and aware, centered, balanced and calm..

1. *Take in a nice, deep breath*
2. *Coming fully into your body*
3. *Integrating this process fully into your body as you begin to move and stretch*
4. *Getting ready to open your eyes, remembering everything you need to know*
5. *Eyes open . . . awake and aware*

Severe Social Anxiety

by Marion Robb

Once upon a time there was a princess and when she was born the nation rejoiced, and her family rejoiced. However, as with all life, there were dangers in the kingdom, some large, some small, and some so tiny as to be no risk at all, but her father the King was very determined that nothing should harm the merest hair on the head of his tiny daughter. And so the King and the Queen built for their daughter a beautiful gilded cage. And it was the most beautiful structure in the land, full of toys and light and games and love. That's right. Within the confines of her dwelling, there were cushions and fountains, and beautiful ornaments of glass in the cage, flowers and cakes and silks and satins on every surface you could see, of every color under the rainbow. And in her cage with her was a beautiful little bird, a bird which sang and spoke and whistled. Through the cage would waft the softest of warm breezes, and the gentlest kiss of the sun on her skin, but on the gate of the cage were 3 large locks, not to keep the Princess in, but to keep the world out. And the Princess kept the keys right round her neck on a very heavy golden chain. And sometimes it felt as if those keys were as heavy as rocks.

And so the first lesson that the Princess learned that the world must be a very dangerous place, and that the people within it were not to be trusted.

As the years went by and the Princess grew older and bigger and stronger, the bars on the cage stopped seeming like a cage and started to seem like a protection. But every day into the cage came a teacher to teach her some lessons, and some school friends to keep her company. And the Princess was very aware that as she was the King's daughter, she had to be on her very best behavior at all times. She had to show everyone the very best of manners and do everything as best as she possibly could. And so the second lesson the Princess learned was to watch every single little thing she said and did, and to think about any tiny little problem with what she said or did over and over again, until it became so exhausting it became easier just to say nothing at all.

And still the Princess continued to grow, until one day she became a lovely, kind and intelligent young woman. All her teachers had finished their work, and she was bright and lively and fun. But her school friends grew and flourished, and left the cage behind and went out to make their way in the world, with scrapes to the knees, and fallings outs, and arguments, and boyfriends, and jobs, and sometimes making mistakes, and sometimes doing well - because as with all life, it is for living. But the Princess was left behind the bars of her gilded cage, and soon she began to droop a little, and to rattle the bars of her cage, and to look out the window at the life going on around her...and soon some Princes from faraway lands were coming to pay court to the Princess, and to hope for her favor, but she was by this time so restrained, that she decided to shut up. And day and night she remained, silent in this cage. By this time the King and Queen realized their mistake and pleaded with the Princess every day to open the cage and come out, but the Princess just shook her head. And so the Princes didn't get to know the lovely young Princess, and thought her to be very restrained, and sadly left without being able to get to know her at all. And so the third lesson the Princess learned was that if she didn't make an effort to leave the cage, then it was going to become a prison and not a protection. And when she realized this, it felt to the Princess like the keys round her neck had become so heavy it was hardly possible to carry them anymore. And so very carefully she removed them, one by one.

One day, feeling brave, she took the smallest key and tried it in the lock, but it was so old and rusty that it would not turn, and no-one in the Kingdom could get it to open, and a call was put out far and wide to find someone who could release the Princess. And so from the furthest corner of the Kingdom came a wise old fairy, quite the oldest and wisest fairy the Princess had ever seen, and through the bars of the cage she handed the Princess a beautiful box, tied up with golden ribbon, saying "a gift for you Princess"... and in the box was a beautiful bracelet and it was made up of letters and the letters spelled "judgment", and a tiny little golden scale. "What is judgment?" said the Princess... "What does it mean?"

And the fairy said, "When we are little we depend upon our elders to tell us and show us the ways of the world, and so we learn the lessons they teach us.... But sometimes those lessons are misjudged, or misguided, or too severe, and so we are all given a gift as we grow older and that is called "judgment"...we all use judgment every day in making every single decision we think of."

"Think of other people," said the fairy. "Now most of us are really very nice people...everyone knows that nobody is perfect...don't you, that's right? So once we are grown judgment helps us to decide who is a person we want to get to know and who is a person that we don't. Because if we don't use judgment there are two things that could happen... firstly, we might not trust anyone at all and in so doing hurt ourselves and others, because can you imagine how you would feel if nobody trusted you? That's right. And if we don't trust anyone at all, it would become very lonely indeed, and life would be much poorer, for people are the most fascinating and interesting creatures in the world, and they can bring us much joy and love. And the second thing that could happen if we didn't use judgment is that we would trust absolutely everybody with everything and if that was the case you'd soon find yourself giving all your money to someone greedy, or telling the Kingdom's secrets to spies, or other things like that."

"I see," said the Princess, "And what is this other little gift...the scales?"

"Ah," said the fairy, "That is not my second gift to you...that is a gift that you must strive to achieve for yourself...and that is balance, Princess, balance. Balance and calibrate your judgment. Finely tune it, work on it every day to help yourself and allow yourself to make judgments about people – is it fair not to trust that person who has shown you kindness and help, who has never done or said anything to hurt you, or is it better to give them the benefit of the doubt and allow them to become a friend? And every time you work on your balance and judgment it will become easier and easier and easier, until you find it's so enjoyable speaking to new people, learning new things, being accepted, to make the first move by smiling or saying hello...and noticing how so many people respond to that by smiling and saying hello back...and how every time they do your confidence grows and grows, and how easy it becomes to speak to others now, that's right."

The Princess nodded her head, and said, "I see what you

mean", and the smallest lock fell from the cage and landed with a large clatter on the ground. But the Princess still had the problem of thinking about every little thing she said and did until it was so bad, that she almost didn't want to speak to anyone at all.

In her cage with her was a beautiful little bird, a bird which sang and spoke and whistled. But as the bird grew older it was as if it had lost its voice. And its feathers grew dull and its eyes grew sad and it forgot to preen its feathers. But in fact the bird was afraid to sing, it was afraid to speak, in case it said the wrong thing or whistled the wrong tune.

And just before the fairy left, she said, "You better teach that bird to talk, or its lovely voice will never be heard and it won't be able to fly. And everyone knows that it's your responsibility to look after that little bird, don't you?"

The Princess understood at once that if the poor little bird was going to ever be able to fly away from the cage, at the same time as she did, she'd have to teach it to talk. And so every day she practiced with the bird. A word here, a sentence there, a smile and a whistle, an opinion here, an opinion there, and the little bird's voice was so pretty, that soon the King and Queen would take time to listen, then the gardeners, and the milkmaids, and the people in the fields and the traffic wardens and the policemen and the men and the women and the boys and the girls, all smiled to hear the bird singing its song, and to hear the Princess speaking merrily away to the little bird, teaching it slowly and progressively how to speak to her, and to others, and to sit proudly on its perch unafraid to make a cheep, or a word, or a song. And all of them were happy for the little bird, happy to hear it sing, and many of them sang along with it.

One day, the King and the Queen and the Princess invited everyone in the land to come and listen to the beautiful little bird sing, and whistle and speak, which it did beautifully, with only the odd little mistake which nobody would ever have noticed, they were so interested in what the bird was saying and singing and whistling. And the little bird bloomed again right in front of everyone eyes, its feathers grew brighter, it puffed out its chest, its little eyes sparkled with mischief and its song grew louder and louder and louder, and its words grew clearer and clearer and more confident with each one.

At the end of the song, the second lock fell from the cage, and landed with a very loud clatter on the ground, leaving just enough room for the little bird to squeeze between the bars and fly off, first around the room, swooping and diving over the heads of the King and Queen and people, all of whom were clapping and laughing, and then, without a backwards glance, the bird soared off out of the window, out into the beautiful blue sky and towards a new horizon.

Now, the Princess was very glad that she had done a good job for the little bird, but she felt even more frustrated, alone in her cage. So she began to fiddle with the last lock and bash it a bit and hit it and still it would not loosen. The Princess really now wanted to leave her gilded cage and get rid of this last, heavy burden round her neck, so that she could take her place in the world amongst all the people in the land, taking with her new balanced judgment about people, and taking with her the fact that she had found her own voice in helping the little bird free itself from its silence. All that now remained was that last lock, the one requiring her to put the effort in to free yourself now.

And so the princess realized that she would have to be brave and put her whole self into getting free, free from constraint, free from this prison she had locked herself into, and so she pushed, and she shoved and she wore the lock down, little bit by little bit, every day edging further and further out into the world, until one day she simply burst right out of the cage, and was so entranced by the world that she found outside, the colors, the smells, the conversations, the smiles, the arguments, the succcsses, the mistakes (for nothing was ever done or built or achieved without error along the way), the laughter, the fun, and the realization that most of the people in the world were just like her, that she totally forgot her gilded cage and never went back. That's right. And she became aware of new feelings, new excitements, new possibilities and opportunities and realized that you are young, pretty and intelligent and the world is your oyster.

That's right.

Depression – Seed to Flower

by Teya Graves

(use your own preferred induction and deepener)

I wonder if you can use your imagination...to follow everything I say...and just let your conscious thoughts...drift away. For a little while, I wonder if you can imagine that maybe, for some people, life is similar to a growing seed. Can you imagine the life of a seed? It begins...in the bloom of a flower... attracting those who seek the beauty that surrounds that tiny seed.

And after a while, the bloom begins to fade, and it will fall down...down to the loving...mother earth below...where the seed will fall...further down...from the old fallen bloom...into the arms and the depths and the protective darkness of mother earth.

Imagine the darkness...buried deep down below, where no one can see...many seem not to know...or even care.

What must it be like to struggle for life...where no one sees? No one can see but the little seed. The others, who enjoy life above the darkness...just cannot see...so they don't know how it feels...to struggle...to try to find the light...and there are others, buried too...who cannot see...who struggle to grow and find their light...and some...never do.

I wonder if you can imagine now, struggling to find the light. Imagine that as a seed...in this beginning...you were once above the darkness. At one time, you were so high...with your face in the sun, shining bright and feeling strong and happy.

You knew what you liked and what you wanted and you had dreams and goals and plans of your own. It might have been just a little while...or maybe it was a long time ago...and it doesn't really matter when it was...but you know...you can remember a time...when you felt so happy...so hopeful.

You enjoyed the sunshine. You enjoyed the wind on your face. You trusted the winds that blew you in one direction...then another...and one day that wind blew...and you fell. You fell and became buried in another time...and as time passed...and seasons changed... others moved around you, some seeming...to not even know you were there, buried in darkness, struggling to grow, alone.

And I wonder now, if you can connect to that darkness and feeling of being alone. I wonder if you know what it's like...to ask for what you want...or request changes for the things you don't want....but it seems as if you are not heard at all...and you feel more alone and you just relax in the darkness for a while...waiting for the sun and the light...to find its way to you...

and I wonder if maybe, in that quiet darkness...you can create your own growth...a little now... while still in that dark, safe, quiet place. Just a little now. Feel yourself, stretch a little. Grow a little stronger and believe and understand...that soon, you will see the light.

Just imagine, as you grow...that the light, above the darkness is waiting...waiting quietly...just for you. Know that you are safe and secure. Imagine that you can believe...how nice it will feel...to sense the warmth of the sun on your face...and to trust the blowing wind again...because you will soon be stronger than you ever were before.

And just as that tiny seed wants to grow...toward the light...just imagine your roots...expanding and growing into mother earth now...as she holds...and surrounds...and nurtures you. And as you feel those roots growing and extending down...your heavy legs and your feet...I want you to move the toes on your **left foot**, just a little...as you feel connected to mother earth now.

Wonderful, and relax your toes as you relax deeper now. It feels so good to know you can just stretch a little as you grow stronger and as you drift and float...in the silence...between the sounds of my voice.

Now imagine the strong roots...begin to grow down into mother earth...from your right foot now. Feel the deep hug...of mother earth now...as she holds...and surrounds ...and nurtures you...feel your roots growing down...as you move your **right** toes, just a little...

Wonderful, and relax your toes...as you connect to that gravitational pull of mother earth...and relax deeper.

> ***(Deepener if needed)*** Allow your gentle breaths in...and out...to relax you more...as you focus only on my voice. All other thoughts and sounds can just dissolve and drift away for a little while as you relax and let go of any tensions.

> ***(Bring up a little if needed)*** Take a deep breath of air and focus on my voice. You are not going to sleep. You are listening to my voice and you are focused your success.

I want you to just imagine now...that your arms and legs are stretching and growing longer...as you are growing stronger and thinking about what it might be like...to one day...poke your head up, out of the darkness. Growing and stretching and relaxing, becoming more open...and stronger...in your mind and body. Feel your own desire, to be in the light that you hope for...one day soon.

And as your desire grows...and as you are growing stronger now... just think about the light, above the darkness...while you rest quietly now.

Think about or imagine...how every tiny seed knew...that in order to grow... it needed to be dropped in dirt...covered in darkness...and it had to struggle and survive...and to finally decide to grow stronger and reach out to the light. It took determination...and strong will to survive...to grow.

When you are finally tired of the darkness...and ready to move into the light...it will be your own decision to grow yourself stronger.

You are here today, because you want to get better. You want to get stronger. You want to focus on your success. Yes, I think you do.

Take a deep...lung-filling breath of air...as you feel yourself grow stronger now...while in this dreamy... relaxed and confident state. And when you ready to move on...and grow into the light...and grow stronger, just raise a finger on one hand so I know this is what you want.

Thank you. I see, that you are ready and willing to grow stronger. Give yourself that all −important permission to focus on your success now.

I would like you to look up now, **with your eyelids still**

closed...Get a picture in your mind of the light filtering through the darkness, beckoning you to come and feel warm.

Now wait a moment, before you push through that last layer of darkness, and move into the light. See each stone or clump of dirt, above you that has held you down.

What obstacles have been in your way? Are some of the clumps of dirt, ideas about not being...

(Use the client's own words as much as possible)

Good enough...smart enough...pretty enough...etc.

Do some of those clumps or rocks represent names you called yourself... or past failures at things you wanted to achieve but did not?

Maybe you see people who told you hurtful things...and those people or statements held you down in the darkness.

Maybe you see your own feelings as a barrier that held you down. What do those hurtful and heavy feelings look like? What do they feel like?

Tell me what you see...What held you in the darkness? What kept you down?

(Thank you for telling me about that)

See it all now. See those thoughts...and feelings...and attachments to the darkness...See them in the stones and the dirt and feel it in the heaviness.

Feel yourself, firmly grounded and growing stronger...as you push past those barriers...as you feel determined...to push through them...and as you get closer to the light...look around and see what else you see...Who has stood by, waiting and hoping for your return? In some cases... it might even be the same person that said hurtful things...as well as others.

Who has encouraged and supported your growth...and now that you are peeking...into the light...this person...is now smiling at you and so proud of you...and so impressed with your great strength ...because they know the strength it took for you...to make the choice...to begin to rise above the darkness...and although in some ways...it is all fresh and new for you, and it seemed so hard...there are people who love you...and have been waiting for you...and will gladly be there for you...as you continue to grow lighter...and taller...and stronger...and brighter...and happier now.

And as you pull yourself up into the light...and focus on what is good...and bright...and positive in your life...

Look at the dirt and the challenges below you...look at the burdens you pushed aside so easily...when you grew yourself stronger. Grow yourself bigger...and stronger... than any challenge.

All darkness...dirt...heaviness and challenges...are simply there for you to have power over...to overcome...to grow yourself...stronger...wiser...and more able to meet the next challenge...with confidence and more and more inner strength and self-respect... and self-love.

I wonder if you might look around...and find yourself in a most beautiful garden now. Look around...and see the others who are with you...maybe you can even get a sense of their growing challenges. See the burdens that once buried them.

226

Who surpassed the burdens and who still looks heavy and weighted down? Who do you see that is strong like a mighty oak...or beautiful...like a perfect rose...do the weeds look bad...or are they just another challenge...to be cast aside?

We all spend time in darkness...some find the light...some grow into strength...some grow into beauty...some become challenges for others and some...never...come into the light...to dance and play with the living.

You have made the choice to come into the light. You have surpassed your burdens and darkness. You can see the gifts and the challenges of others and you can choose...who you will dance with...and when.

You are bright. You are strong. You are beautiful. You are the light. The light is within you. It always has been within you...hiding beneath the darkness and now you have risen above that darkness and it feels right. It feels good. It feels strong. It feels new and permanent...and you want to share that light.

It's a bright and beautiful day. You are standing tall and strong as you have pulled yourself up and out of the darkness. You no longer focus on obstacles or challenges. You focus on what is beautiful around you. You focus on the light...and the good...and you focus on solutions and goals and working toward making yourself strong enough to surpass, any obstacle.

You know that you used to feel held down in the darkness...and you know what it was...that held you down...and now you have the great pleasure of knowing that nothing...can ever...hold you down again.

You have grown and you are growing still...stronger and more confident and happier with all that is around you and all that is within you...that made you who you are...and who you are...is beautiful... confident and strong.

Hold your head high...and your shoulders back...and feel how much taller you are...as you take a deep breath of air and let it out slowly...admiring who you are...as every breath relaxes you deeper.

Sense only the beauty of this new birth. See only the strength and the gentleness and the desire and the passion to continue to grow stronger now. Desire...more inner strength. It's OK to love yourself. You are worthy of self-love. You are worthy of self-respect. Embrace it.

Allow the darkness of the past to stay in the past. Allow the darkness to be known...for what it truly is. It is just a story, from the past...that brought you to where you are now. The past doesn't exist. The future does not exist. The past is just a story. The future is just a story, yet untold. The only **truth** is this moment now...And **this** moment now...and this moment **now**.

Everything before and after **this moment now**...is just a story. Live in the present...here and now. Remember and learn from the past. Plan for and dream of...a positive future. Correct and continue when challenges occur.

Commit yourself...to your growth. Commit to growing stronger and happier and wiser and healthier...in your body...and your mind...and your spirit.

Allow all the muscles of your body to just soften and relax. Drift deeper and deeper into a blissful state of hypnosis, while staying focused on my voice.

I want you to focus, for a moment now on the inside of your brain. Just imagine...the inside of your wonderful brain, with all the work that is done there. See the pathways...and electrical impulses...and the deeper levels of workings...down to the hypothalamus...the power center of your brain...that creates all those feel good chemicals...that help you to move...and to sleep...and to have more energy when needed.

The hypothalamus is responsible for hormone production...to govern body temperature...thirst... hunger...sleep...moods...sex drive...and the release of other hormones in the body. You tell your hypothalamus, both consciously and subconsciously to create the most proper amounts of hormones...and chemicals...at the best times.

Tell your brain that you want to feel happier...more excited about life. Tell the deepest part of your wonderful brain...that you want a more balanced release...of the feel good...natural chemicals...of serotonin...dopamine...and the chemical Oxytocin...which is usually released...during long...warm ...safe hugs...but can be released any time...you sense hugging and loving yourself.

Tell your brain to create the healthiest...natural chemicals...and hormones...for your best health and your best happiness and your best levels of understanding of the goodness...of the world around you.

Focus on your success. Focus on what you want, not on what you don't want. When you have a thought that does not support your best success, say, "Cancel that thought," and replace it with a new, better thought.

You will sleep very well at night...when you are supposed to sleep...and you will wake up feeling more refreshed and strengthened, every day. You feel strong and happy...looking for the light...and conquering any obstacles...that merely help you...to grow stronger...and you find more pride and confidence...within you. This is what you want. This is what you asked for. This is for you.

Unpacking the Back Pack

by Shannon King

A script to help relieve anxiety and sleeplessness

Once upon a time...there was a young boy...and this little boy was full of curiosity and joy...he just wanted to play and have fun. He loved to play outside and at the beach (or client's choice). He would run and jump, and play with his dogs (or client's favorite animal or toy). He would love to walk along the ocean beach and smell the clean, salty ocean air. He loved to do whatever he wanted to do...which was to play and have fun.

One day, this little boy was given a backpack...it was a big backpack, with lots of pockets and compartments...lots of spaces to put anything in the backpack he wanted. There were pockets with zippers, and open compartments that you could look right into. There were even a few secret compartments that only the little boy knew about...places he could hide the things he wanted to hide. And the little boy was so excited....he began his collection of stuff.

Each day, he would wake up in the morning, so excited because he had so many things to collect...there was playing and having fun to be done! So each day, the little boy would put on his backpack and start his day. At first, he collected things he really liked...he would put them into the open spaces in his backpack. They gave him such joy; he wanted to see them every time he looked into his backpack. His backpack began to fill up...but all the good stuff that made him happy and joyful...never made his backpack heavy.

231

Eventually, the little boy found something that he wasn't quite sure about...it didn't make him feel as happy as all the good stuff in his backpack and he didn't really want it mixed in with his good stuff...so he put it into a different pocket...one of the pockets he didn't have to look at a lot. And the little boy continued to collect his stuff.

As the little boy got a little older...he carried his backpack with him everywhere...and he still loved to play and have fun...and collect his stuff. He put the good stuff he collected with his other good stuff...in the open spaces because he loved to look at this stuff whenever he looked into his backpack. And along the way, he collected more stuff that didn't make him as happy as all the good stuff...and he collected stuff that made him sad...and he collected stuff that made him feel bad...and he didn't know why he kept this stuff...and he really didn't want this stuff that made him feel sad or bad...so he put this sad and bad stuff into different pockets. He put the stuff that was just so-so sad into pockets that he had to purposely look into to see the stuff in there...and he put the really sad stuff into zippered pockets so he couldn't see the stuff unless he opened the pocket and looked inside. And he noticed the good stuff never made his backpack feel heavy, but every piece of sad or bad stuff made his backpack heavier and heavier.

As the little boy grew older and went to school...where he found lots of good stuff to collect and put into his backpack...and he found some stuff that wasn't so good. But he was so used to collecting everything he found, he kept this stuff too, even though it made him sad or feel bad. He continued to put these things into the pockets he didn't want to look into. Some of the stuff he even put into the secret pockets so he never had to look at it. And he forgot about it.

But it made his backpack heavier and heavier.

And the young boy grew older and went to junior high, and high school...and eventually he grew into a man. And all the time, he carried his backpack with him. And he collected good stuff...stuff that made him happy...that made him feel like the little boy that played and had fun. And when he looked at his good stuff and played and had fun he felt wonderful! He felt relaxed and peaceful. He also continued to collect the stuff that wasn't so good...and because he didn't want it to make him feel sad or bad...he would hide it away in the closed and secret pockets of his backpack...and the backpack became so heavy...so heavy that it started to hurt him to carry it. It hurt his body...and it hurt his mind...because he knew he was carrying this bad stuff around. But he didn't remember what it was anymore because he had hidden it inside his backpack where he didn't have to look at it.

One day, when the little boy was a grown man...he realized his backpack was so heavy, it hurt him so bad to carry it...he didn't want to carry it anymore. He still loved it...but it no longer made him happy because it weighed him down. He couldn't have as much fun because he couldn't move as much...he couldn't sleep because even in bed it weighed heavily on his heart and mind. He couldn't do the things he loved as much because he was tired...and his body hurt...and his mind hurt...and his heart hurt.

So the grown man decided it was time to clean out his backpack. He had no idea what he would find, since it had been a long time since he had looked at some of the stuff he had hidden away. Since the man loved the (*favorite place*) so much, he decided it would make him happy to go to the (*favorite place*)...so, he took his backpack and went to the (*favorite place*).Just being there made him feel happy...and relaxed...and safe...and he knew it was the perfect place to go through his backpack.

So, very slowly, he opened his backpack...and at first he saw all the good stuff in his backpack...and it made him happy and peaceful. He carefully gathered all the good stuff and put it to the side because he was going to keep it. Then, taking a deep breath...he started to look into the other pockets...and as he started to look at the stuff he had put in there...as he looked at it he remembered how it had made him feel...and he realized he no longer felt sad or bad...all that old stuff was from the past...it no longer meant anything to him...and he could just take it all out of the backpack and throw them into the ocean...and he sat for a while and watched that stuff float away. Watched it float farther and farther away...growing smaller until it completely disappeared...That wasn't so bad!

Taking another deep breath...and feeling more confident than before...he unzipped the first zippered pocket that he hadn't looked into for a long time...and as he looked at the stuff...he realized it no longer was useful to him...it didn't make him happy and it no longer had the power to make him sad...he could just take it out and throw it into the ocean. If he found something that was useful to him...and added to his happiness and peace, then he would rub it in the sand and rinse it in the ocean so it looked new and put it to the side with his good stuff.

Pocket after pocket...he went through each pocket and took out all the bad stuff...knowing he didn't need it...and he threw it in the ocean. After going through all the zippered pockets...he went on to the secret pockets. He was now very curious to look into these secret pockets where he put things he never wanted to look at...because he knew he had collected all that stuff in the past and he was actually kind of excited because he knew he could simply throw it into the ocean if it was no longer useful. And if he could find a purpose for it and it made him happy...he could rub it in the sand and rinse it in the ocean and make it new so it fit with his good stuff. Pocket by pocket, he went through all the stuff he had collected...and the bad stuff that was no longer useful...he threw into the ocean and watched it float away...watched it get smaller and smaller...floating farther and farther away...until he couldn't see it any longer.

Surprised, he realized he had nothing left that wasn't in his good stuff pile...everything he had left was useful and had a purpose...and made him happy...gave him joy and peace...And he collected all the good stuff and put it back into his backpack, in the open spaces so he could look at it anytime he wanted. He stood up and picked up his backpack...and as he raised it off the sand it seemed to just fly up into the air it was so light. When he put it on his back, he couldn't even feel the weight of the good stuff in his backpack...it was so light...and it made him feel so good. He felt good. His body felt good. His mind felt good. His heart felt good.

And that night, for the first time in a long time...when he went to sleep, he was so comfortable and calm and relaxed...he fell right to sleep and slept soundly all night long...waking in the morning, refreshed and relaxed. He knew that because his backpack was now filled with good stuff and not bad stuff he had to carry about, he would sleep soundly every night and wake up feeling wonderfully good... so that he could play and have fun!

The Magic Box

by Camilla Edborg

This script outline is used for letting go of fears and other negative feelings. It would be very beneficial if you use the script, The Strength Secret, on page 252 first, a powerful combination.

There are probably some old fears and misunderstandings from the past, you know...old feelings from which you really do not benefit. Experience provides you with wisdom and learning, giving you inner strength, but perhaps the feelings caught in them aren't needed anymore.

Well, let me tell you about a great thing here, there is a beautiful box slightly behind you. This great box is actually quite marvelous. As I open it for you, all parts of you, (*enhance voice*) and I am now talking to all parts of (*name of client*) both body and subconscious, can release all negative or dark feelings that harm you in any way...just let them go so that I can help them have a chance to feel good instead...

You see, this box is like a magnet to your negative feelings, or feelings that don't even belong to you and in a moment I will open it, and you can now allow yourself to get rid of hate, anger, anxiety, guilt, fear, all feelings we all have felt at one point or another in life...even jealousy, hatred, envy, disgust...all of it...

Once you let go of all the negative feelings and all cell memories can let go, you will be able to be healed...fantastically, easily and in a wonderful way.

So, in a moment, I will open the box and you can just let all negative emotions pour out and go straight into that box...are you ready? (*wait for yes*)

I am opening this beautiful box now...simply allow yourself this treat, *feel*...you can now just *feel* how all those negative feelings (it's just like a magnet!) flow away from you... away from your body...away easily moving into this marvelous box. All pain in the cell memories can now dissipate, let go, as your mind and body realizes that it was just a learning experience and it can now be healed.

I will let you have some time to get ALL of it out. All pain in the cell memories that are not needed anymore. You can let me know with a finger signal or a nod or your voice when you are completely done.

When client lets you know...verify that all unwanted and unnecessary feelings have been released and allow for more processing time if needed.

Now, just imagine a bright, golden light...let this light shine through...and you notice, the rays of light reach right into that box and start to dissolve and transform those emotions using this loving light... how wonderful ... all emotions that were so dark are now being beautifully dissolved and transformed by this light turning into wonderful positive energy....So quickly...so effectively. *(wait some time for this to happen... some clients can tell when it is done)*

The box is now empty and the transformed light emotions can, if it is for the best and if they truly belong to you, go back and help you, or they can follow the light rays up... where they will be taken care of in a beautiful safe way.

I will now close the box. But that wonderful light is now changing slightly, you can sense the healing light, the love it feels for you...so feel how it gently fills all the empty spaces inside of you with love, light and healing...all places inside of you, even if some negative feelings have been hiding...they can now transform to light...

Can you feel it ?

(If no, then there are several heavy ego blocks in the way, just continue, as it will help anyway.)

Let's allow the light to fill you up entirely so that you can feel wonderful, and let me know when this is completed.

Now close all entrances inside of you and keep this light inside of you, and we will let the light slowly withdraw, leaving just this wonderful, enhanced, wiser and happier, *(incorporate how the client wants to feel afterwards)* new, amazing you...

...the You that now has the possibility to see things from another view, another perspective that will help enhance your life experiences in many ways.

Chapter 9   Weight and Eating Issues

Majestic Closet

by Maria Sideris

I invite you to visualize or imagine the grandest mansion you have ever seen in your life. You feel this mansion provides you with shelter, safety, and peace of mind. You sense like you belong there. You start to walk down a gorgeous path to the grand entrance of the mansion. As you stroll towards its inviting doors you feel a sense of peace. I invite you to allow all your senses to come alive as you may smell the aroma of the flowers that surround and embellish the gardens along the path and mansion. You might notice their vibrant colours of luscious reds, playful pinks, peaceful yellows and healing greens. You may even hear the sweet songs from birds overhead showering you with their melody. Allow yourself to feel the warm, orange kisses of the sunrays tickling your skin. Taste the freshness of the air as the soft wind envelops you in love, guiding you as you stroll down further towards the door.

Waking down towards the doors of the mansion now...10...9...8...7...6...5...half way there...4...3...2...1...

You reach the doors, open them and walk in. Here you notice a grand foyer with hallways leading to rooms. You walk down the hallway instinctively knowing where to go to find your room. Once you get to it you walk in and notice it's the closet of your dreams. This closet is filled with rows and rows of beautiful and dignified clothes. This closet is majestic. There are shelves and shelves of shoes boots, and purses to match every outfit. You notice racks of bikinis, bathing suits, nightgowns, pyjamas and the most luxurious, sexy lingerie you have ever seen.

You want to try on the clothes in this majestic closet, so you reach over to grab the first article of clothing. It's the outfit you have always imagined yourself wearing when you look your sexiest and most beautiful. You peel it off the hanger to put it on, except you notice it doesn't fit. It doesn't fit because you are suddenly aware that you are all covered up and weighed down by layers and layers of old dingy, worn out, thick, abrasive, musty smelling clothes. Allow yourself now to feel the full capacity of how all these layers of old unneeded clothes are weighing you down. All these layers are keeping you from wearing all the new gorgeous clothes hanging in all these rows and rows in this majestic closet. Feel how it feels when you cannot wear what you want. Feel what it feels like when you cannot fit into these perfect sized clothes tailored made just for your gorgeous slim, trim and healthy body that is presently being enclosed and weighed down by all that that no longer serves you.

I invite you to own these feelings of unnecessary heaviness, and now look up and notice the mirror in the closet...look at it...look deep into your own eyes shining brightly back at you and in your mind...repeat after me:

I now realize I am responsible for my body, my health, and my peace of mind. I now realize and accept that I am responsible for allowing any negative words, actions or thoughts to enter my mind, my body and my soul. I accept that I may choose at times to eat in order to fill any voids of love, loneliness, low self-worth and unfulfilled dreams or negative thoughts and emotions. These old beliefs and behaviour patterns have layered my body with layers and layers of unhealthy, unnecessary weight. I now choose to let go, release any need I had to use food to feel whole. I lovingly release all my past beliefs, behaviours, patterns and any negative conditioned responses I had with food. I know I have the power to be all that I can be. My mind is my tool to live in perfect health and peace of mind. I am in total control of my mind. I am in total control of every thought, word and action I take both in my conscious and unconscious states.

Now look into that mirror and visualize or imagine yourself peeling off, shedding or tearing off all those layers of old dingy, worn out, thick, abrasive, musty smelling clothes you are layered in. With each layer you tear off, peel off, or shed, you are removing old negative patterns, of self-abuse...negative self-talk...and unworthiness. You tear off and rid yourself of negative behaviours and criticisms that have weighed you down. You no longer need to hide under all these layers. With every layer you shed, you let go and release all your past beliefs and negative conditioned responses.

Focus on my voice and in your mind repeat after me: with each layer I shed...tear off... or peel off...I remove, release, and let go of all that no longer serves me in living a life of health and peace of mind.

I invite you to now notice all those layers that are there piled up on the floor. You are now free of all the unneeded layers of all that weighed you down, and now you are left in your perfect form. I invite you to take look in the mirror again and visualize or imagine your body in its perfect form...free from all the excess it has been carrying around.

Beside you is a big canvas laundry bag labeled: ideas, beliefs and habits that don't serve me any longer. Throw into it every layer of those old dingy, worn out, thick, abrasive, musty smelling clothes. Dispose of all those layers made up of old negative patterns of self-abuse, negative self-talk, and unworthiness. Throw into the canvas bag everything you need and feel you must get rid of so you can continue on with your real life.

Now that you have disposed of all that no longer serves you, you face the mirror and repeat in your mind after me: I now know that holding on to anything in my past just weighs me down so I let go, release and forgive. I have removed and stepped out of all these unneeded unnecessary layers that have weighed me down in the past. I have rid of them for good, releasing myself to be lighter both inside and out.

Allow yourself to fully embrace your perfectly healthy, slim, trim body reflecting back into your bright eyes. Let go and allow yourself to feel once again with all your senses. Looking at the mirror, you might notice it has bright lights that flash in congratulation and to the rhythm of the celebratory music which fills the closet. Allow yourself to sense the vibration of the music as it travels into your core, brewing up a feeling of euphoria. You may even find yourself dancing and singing. You might even notice a swell of tears forming or maybe spilling out of your eyes. That's okay, these are tears of joy vibrating from the love you have for yourself, for you have finally embraced your true self.

I invite you now to pick the most gorgeous outfit you can find in the closet, be aware of the textures, patterns and colours of the fabrics...starting from the sexy lingerie, now move on to the clothes...next, you choose the most amazing shoes and complimenting purse and coat. You put on the final touches of make-up and accessories then look back into the mirror and visualize or imagine the complete package. You look beautiful, dignified, healthy, slim and trim. You look and are majestic.

You may feel a sense of pride or empowerment now. Allow yourself to feel the strength that rises up from deep inside you, knowing that you can accomplish whatever you set your mind on. I invite you to now grab that canvas bag and walk out the closet, then straight out the back door of the mansion. You head for a fire pit in the back yard. You go up to it and throw in the fire that bag which is filled with all that no longer serves you. I invite you to stand back at a safe distance to watch it burn. Observe as it is ablaze and dissipates into nothingness, releasing you to move forward.

You might want to say to yourself as you watch it burn: I completely and tenderly forgive myself first and then all others that I need to, in order to move forward with my life. With a peaceful mind I now embrace my healthy, trim, slim body and self which has been waiting patiently to step out and live, breathe, and belong in my life.

Goldilocks and the Small Plate

by Toni Macri Reiner

Weight loss, smaller portion, healthy eating script. This is a story I use in the middle of a weight loss session, interjecting it between direct suggestions and ego strengthening.

One day, Goldilocks went for a walk in the forest. It was a beautiful day...the trees were beginning to change colors...the leaves, in shades of reds, yellows and oranges were so beautiful. The air was crisp and clean, even invigorating! Goldilocks was so thoroughly enjoying her brisk pace that it was quite some time until she realized she had walked a long way. She checked her stomach and realized that she was hungry. But she was far from home...what could she eat that would help her stomach feel satisfied? It was at this point when she spied, in the distance, the house of the three bears.

Goldilocks knew that the Bear family was out for their daily brisk walk, but since the bears always welcomed her into their home, she was sure they wouldn't mind if she stopped for a small bite to eat. Pushing open the door to their charming cottage, she was very happy to see the table set for a meal.

The first chair she came to was Papa Bear's heavy, massive mountain of a chair! It was so big that she immediately felt overwhelmed. As she looked at Papa's huge plate of food, food that was heavy, greasy & full of fat, she imagined how sick she would feel if she ate that unhealthy food. And such large portions...no wonder Papa was SO big!

Quickly she moved away from that large plate of food & heavy chair.

Next she sat in Mama Bear's chair. And while it wasn't quite as large as Papa's chair, it was still too heavy for her and made her feel very small. Mama's plate was a bit smaller than Papa's but still it, too, was excessive for her. The food on the plate was just pretending to be healthy. She could tell it had hidden fats, sugars & salts just waiting to make her feel bloated for some time after she ate it. The portions were still too big for a girl of her size.

Goldilocks quickly removed herself from the sight of that plate which was holding oversized portions of unhealthy food.

Next, she settled into Baby Bear's chair. Ahhhh, now this felt just right! This chair helped her to feel slim in all the right places, not heavy like the other chairs. She was so happy to see Baby's small plate, small portion sizes and his glass of fresh, clean water. The food in front of her looked so healthy: fresh, nutrient dense food, lots of vibrant colors, veggies & healthy protein. Just looking at those foods made her feel good, knowing that 30 minutes after she ate she would feel healthy, satisfied & happy.

This is how Goldilocks wanted to eat whenever her stomach told her it needed some nourishment so she began to enjoy the beautiful meal...eating slowly, relishing each and every bite as she chewed the food thoroughly. She found that it because the food was so healthy, she quickly became fulfilled and satisfied...because less is more when you find just the right amount for yourself.

And from now on, you choose to eat just as Goldilocks and Baby Bear do... enjoying smaller portions of fresh nutrient-dense food from healthy sources...and drinking plenty of fresh, clean water.

Weight Loss Plateaus

by Linda Roan

Find out what successes the client has had in the past and incorporate below........

And, from time to time, you reach a plateau with your weight release but just as you had the persistence to overcome other obstacles in your life, you persevere with your meal plans and exercise and you shed weight safely and easily knowing you are successful in your weight release goals. And you are successful because you take the time for yourself because your goals are important...Muscle weighs more than fat...sometimes your body retains water, sometimes you reach a plateau; sometimes your weight may shift up and down but you persist with your weight loss goals undeterred because you know that by continuing to eat vegetables, fruits, lean proteins and low calorie, fibrous carbs and pursuing a variety of movement and exercise every day you have more energy... you easily reach your weight loss goal and maintain it. With persistence and determination, you reach your weight loss goal and maintain the healthy weight that you desire for the rest of your life, proud of all your accomplishments...renewing your commitment to your weight loss goals...

You easily and comfortably work through plateaus...checking in with all the inner wisdom you have gained...easily recognizing and sensitive to your body's signals...knowing with your inner wisdom...when you've had sufficient to eat...knowing that you can enjoy a wide variety of vegetables and fruits and lean, smaller portions of proteins and healthy carbs...you have eliminated the empty calories of sugary, salty, greasy food and high calorie, sweet juices and alcohol, drinking alcohol reduces the body's fat burning abilities...because you enjoy drinking refreshing water...you release more and more fat cells and toxins, the more water you drink the more weight you release...renewing your commitment to your weight loss goals...

Knowing there are many choices of low calorie foods...succulent berries full of fiber, carrots, apples...for nibbling and crunching...seeking out new recipes, tantalizing your taste buds, bringing discovery in, letting dullness out...knowing that plateaus can be overcome, remembering your successes of the past...*(Hypnotist: insert what you've been told about client successes)*...feeling those successes now in every cell of your body, really feeling and remembering.

And whenever you crave any sugary, greasy...*(unhealthy choices)*foods you feel hot and prickly and release all desire for sugary, greasy...*(unhealthy choices)*...foods. Whenever you picture a cool, blue sky you feel calm and comfortable and desire a fruit or a vegetable...renewing your commitment to your weight loss goals...

Begin to tune into your body's signals as you are now ...recognizing...responding...understanding and assessing your body's hunger signals...are you truly hungry?

Sense the difference between hunger and emotion ...recognizing and acknowledging the difference between hunger and emotion...responding, making time for the things you love to do...easily making wise choices...keeping in touch with your body's wisdom...taking the time...and

247

checking in with your body...knowing when to eat, understanding the body needs regular fuel like a car...you would never allow your car to totally run out of fuel...when you eat too little your body puts the brakes on your metabolism...You are now remaining satisfied with small, regular portions of foods, healthy snacks, balancing your metabolism...a regular metabolism that allows you to easily release weight...as you are now renewing your commitment to your weight loss goals

Having a filling snack before socializing, having a plan before you go, drinking refreshing water, releasing all desire for sugary drinks or alcohol, planning meals in advance, in whatever way works best for you, adapting, changing as you change, changing movement, changing exercising, changing meal plans, exploring new tastes, choosing a wider variety of fresh vegetables and fruits, open to making adjustments, listening to your body's signals...knowing what to eat and how much...making smart choices...staying satisfied...and always, always, every day, having small snacks prepared...wherever you go...releasing all desire to overeat or become hungry...planning easily and comfortably...renewing your commitment to your weight loss goals...

It takes twice as much energy to burn fat, realizing that any extra movements you can add to your day increases the amount of energy expended...stretch, warm up, vigorously exercise, cool down...understanding your body's signals. Adding and increasing movement, changing exercises, enjoying action as you successfully move through a plateau...increasing movement, finding things you love to do...releasing more and more unnecessary fat...as you renew your commitment to your weight loss goals...

And always, always...every day...practicing self care, filling up the spaces in your heart with activities that give you pleasure...enjoying the people with whom you spend time ...acknowledging your accomplishments...recognizing moments of personal growth...building emotional strength...knowing that what others say or do is about them...their fears, their beliefs, their experiences...be yourself, stay true to yourself, all that you need is within you, all the love, all the understanding...is within you...you can do this...you can reach and stay at your goal weight, healthy, lean and slim...renewing your commitment to your weight loss goals...

Imagine yourself surrounded by tempting food, imagine yourself walking away, feeling proud, full of self respect and self worth...LOCK IN THAT FEELING... PRESS TOGETHER YOUR THUMB AND INDEX FINGER AND SAY TO YOURSELF I AM PROUD OF ALL THAT I HAVE ACCOMPLISHED as you renew your commitment to your weight loss goals...

Chapter 10 Transformation

Ego-Strengthening and Removal of Blocks

by Camilla Edborg

Start with a relaxation induction. Once a light trance has been established, ask the client to build a bubble or pyramid of protection around her, so that no negative energies can get in, keeping them completely safe and secure. (This has also helped the ego part or subconscious to open up more as they notice you take care of their wellbeing...) Ask client to fill the protective strong bubble/pyramid (or whatever client has chosen) with light so that he/she even can breathe this wonderful light as it strengthen him/her with every breath (light is especially important if night terror is one of the issues).

Wait until the client has built everything, then continue with deepening...until they have attained the desired level of relaxation or hypnosis, depending on how you work.

In hypnosis or a meditative state, you can choose to do one or more of following. If it is possible, time wise, you can do all of it in one session. However, make sure to include the strengthening process as some point.

The Strength Secret

I use different approaches for strengthening the self, depending on the client and the needs, but I always use my own addition. This is a great tool as it helps the person to relax more and see things more positive in life. In the end it also helps the person to be more tolerant to others which can help relationships in general, and therefore helps the client.

(One of my favorites is looking in the mirror. It has helped some of my clients who find it hard to love themselves.)

You have done such a great job that I will tell you a secret...and it will make positive changes for you. Change how you perceive things in a very positive way. It will help you understand so much easier....help you in so many ways...so as you rest comfortably...I will tell you:

Did you know that ALL mistakes ONLY are learning opportunities...and you know... that means that EVERY learning opportunity is an experience that gives you knowledge in one way or the other...for instance, if you made a mistake, afterwards you KNOW that's not the way to do it, and you can find another way. With every experience you gain knowledge, right? With every knowledge you gain wisdom...and wisdom is really strength, inner STRENGTH. It is so helpful to know this...

And this secret and this knowledge will be part of you now, be part of your subconscious mind and how you manage, react and feel things....a tool just to help you.

The most wonderful thing is, that every learning experience is actually a PERSONAL strengthening tool...YOUR personal strengthening tool...that you can use anytime...

This is true simply because every experience, no matter if it is working out perfectly or not, makes you wiser...Every situation makes you wiser.....How wonderful is that?!

So ALL experience in life is actually ALL strengthening knowledge as you NOW know HOW to look at it... from a new LEARNING perspective...

This means too, that during the years you have ALREADY gathered so many experiences...good and perhaps what can be considered bad, but all ones which did in fact teach you something too, giving you wisdom and strengths...inner strengths...

So from now on you KNOW that all new situations are to be experienced to gain inner strengths, and you can even smile inside at that...and look at it from a constructive learning perspective.

Imagine your NEW response, now...OK, what can I learn from THIS?...almost like a quiz...always from a positive standpoint. Even old situations that seem to be on-going and stuck...perhaps a new look at it from another perspective, with your new tools can be useful...this new perspective...

This information will sink deeply within you and stay forever, to help you. So from now on, allow yourself to feel how wonderful it is to actually understand this...

Everything is just opportunities to learn and develop strength and wisdom, and everything is okay. There is

ALWAYS a positive learning experience to be made ... an strength to gain...

What an opportunity this gives YOU...YOU can CHOOSE how to REACT...and of course, now that you KNOW that it will be a further addition to your strengths, it helps you... every time you are in a new situation, with this understanding, you can easily see that HOW you REACT has changed in a constructive, curious and positive way...STEPPING OUT of the situation and looking at it from your new perspective...calm inside, knowing that it is an experience to be understood and that it strengthens you, but perhaps you don't always know WHAT until it has played out. And that is ok...calm and secure...

With this new understanding...fear has no place because knowledge and strength have taken its place. Knowledge and strength...in a respectful, loving way...simply wonderful...you can now appreciate yourself...and all of the experiences you already have made....

Another wonderful benefit of this new awareness is that you also now KNOW how others go through this same journey of gaining wisdom and strength...perhaps they just don't know it yet...which means that you have even more understanding...you can let go of irritations that only harm you anyway and you can see the beauty in other's experiences...that it is their journey...their own responsibility

...this you understand...

No matter what situation, what person or anything else...you now KNOW this secret. You can use it...and it helps you so much...You choose to find the positive side to any situation so that it can become a strengthening tool in your life.

Removal of Blocks

These client-centered processes are designed for removal of blocks and harmful emotions and are typically used over more than one session. I use my strengthening process above to prepare the client prior to addressing the blocks.

1. Establish Contact

I would like to talk to the higher self or oversoul of (client's name). *The higher self or wiser part that knows everything and IS PART* (very important it is part of the client) *of the client. Can the subconscious kindly let this wiser part come forward?* (wait for signal fingers or nodding) *Thank you very much.*

2. Easily Removed Blocks

I would like the higher self to scan the body and all energy fields belonging to the client.

There might be some blocks or energies that are not beneficial that can be removed by you right now. Would you be kind and scan the body and energy fields and remove these right away and let me know when it is completed with a yes signal?
(might take 2-5 min)

3. Client's Own Blocks

Now, I would like the higher self to scan the body and all places necessary for energies and blocks that belong to the client and let me know how many there are by sending the information to (client's name*)'s conscious mind, but* (client's name*) will continue to remain in this relaxed mode.*

Or... have the client visualize a white board and see what the higher self writes down.

Write down this number for later, then after removal of external, discuss and talk to these one by one next session. If time, perhaps just take one.

Next session(s):

Ask the higher self to bring forward the most important block to start with. (It is usually a scared ego part that needs help to heal and feel better). Continue with emotions until all blocks are cleared. If time is running out, make sure that you end with a positive script/ending.

Ask what emotion this block is in charge of (can be several, do same exercise below for all). For each block, ask:

- what happened
- how old they are
- would they like to be shown a way to heal and feel better
- are there several of you having the same emotions

When information is gathered try the following example:

I would like to talk to the emotion (hate, fear, etc.) *directly. I ask this emotion to come forward so that I can share some wonderful news.*

Are there any more emotions attached to this emotion?
(If the answer is yes, make sure these emotions are handled
in same session or together with the primary one).

Can you all hear me? (yes or nod of head, finger yes)
otherwise continue anyway after a moment. Some are
reluctant until they have seen what you can do and how.

*I know a very easy and fun way to make you feel better.
Would you like to have a look at it?*   (yes or no answer)

*It is almost a bit of a treasure hunt. You see, there is a
amazing, almost magical energy hidden and when you find
it, and touch it, you will feel fantastic. That's it, easy, isn't
it?*
*So let me now show you how to find it...you see, you will
have to look inside yourself. Pretty cool place to hide. Who
knew?!*

*Well, let's see if you can put your feelings aside and look
inside yourself, in the middle or core of yourself; this is
where you will find this light energy. You put it there
yourself a long time ago, so it is harmless. It belongs to you.
It is you!*

*It is usually shaped like a ball or a crystal wand. I will give
you some time to look for it. Let me know by a yes signal or
nod when you have found it.*

wait a few minutes....*Have you found it?*

NO - *remember to put your feelings on the side, it's in there,*

in the middle of you.
YES - *great, isn't it beautiful?* (yes)... *well it does belongs to you...so simply touch it to open this treasure....*(wait a moment...)

Have you received healing now?
NO - (then they haven't touched it and you need to explain nothing more than healing and some great knowledge will be given -that it is the client's self, nothing can harm them)
YES (feeling great)

Now - I ask the higher self to help this energy to go where it belongs and to incorporate all parts ready in the body and soul the way it should be done. I also ask you to let the information about this be known to the subconscious and body parts involved.

Are there any emotions missed that belonged to this part?
(Sometimes there are anxiety with hate. Make sure to take care of any emotions that were attached to this emotion; you don't want to let the client go feeling anxious.)

Once all emotions for that session are taken care of, make sure to inform the subconscious and the body:

I am now talking to the subconscious and the body.... I am now talking to the subconscious and the body.

Have you been informed that today we have healed (list) emotions ? (yes/no)

I need you to make sure that all parts involved are informed, please make sure to inform the part in charge of routine and control. They need to know that this is healed.

Depending on the situation, you might need to do an exercise to show HOW the new routine shall handle the situation. (This is where the previous strengthening process is useful in already laying the foundation for success.)

Speak directly to Subconsious: *Just to show how he/she can NOW choose to react, let's have a look at a new way.*

Bring forward 2 old and 3 new situations and run through them in the way the client would like to feel and act.

Thank you all for great cooperation. Pleasure to work with you. Goodbye for now.

4.External blocks and energies

I now ask the higher self to perform the same procedure, but this time scanning for external energies, and blocks that <u>do not</u> belong to the client and give us the number.

I talk to all external blocks first. I ask them all to listen to what I have to say and the information they have missed.

Information:
Do you all know that you DO NOT belong to (client's name)? *(Usually NO or unsure answer)*

Well, there is a secret you probably don't know about. It's a special thing that contains information, amazing knowledge and even healing powers. And the funny thing is, it's hidden, and as it happens, I know where. It's a bit of a treasure, really. It's also hidden in a very clever way. Are you interested in finding it? (usually yes)

The clever thing is, YOU, yourself hid it there, and then you forgot. Quite a clever place, too. So, lets go find it!

I want all now (keep in mind xx amount of blocks*) to look inside of yourself, into the core. Into the very center of yourself. There is a hidden energy there. It looks like a crystal ball or crystal wand...it's very beautiful.*

So I am now waiting for all of you to find it and let me know when it is found...so I can tell you about the next step. All of you...bear in mind that you need to put aside all emotions so that they don't block your way of finding it. (Usually 1-2 minutes, some takes longer).

Is there anyone that has NOT found the energy? (yes/no - wait longer if yes*)*
Now to open this ... it's a very easy thing to do, you just touch it...because it is yours...
But you can only open your own...And after that you can ask questions about anything. Pretty cool isn't it?

After they have touched it, they feel really good. I ask if there is anything else they want to know (always NO, otherwise they have not touched it). Make sure they ALL touch it.

Confirm: are they ready to continue their journey, or go back to where they came from with their new knowledge ... to be able to heal and help the body, etc... (yes) Thank them and say goodbye.

Movie of Your Future

by Susan French

For weight loss and fitness goals

It's time to BE THE ROCK STAR IN THE MOVIE OF YOUR LIFE. Let your mind drift down into that wonderful state of mind we call hypnosis. The state of faster, easier learning, the state in which new feelings, thoughts and behaviors are formed. You've been in that state before, so let yourself drift down into it again.

Begin by letting your eyes easily close, when you are ready to receive these new learnings. That's right. Let your eyelids close and can you notice now, how they remember to close more and more tightly, heavier, sleepier, more tightly closed. Can you remember a time when you were awakened from a sound sleep? And it took a moment for you to remember how to open your eyes. For just a moment, they seemed stuck closed, glued shut. That's right. Remember. Or imagine that that could happen. I'm certain you've seen it happen to other people, to babies, to pets, people in the movies or on TV? That moment or reorientation back to awakeness...when it just seems like you can't quite remember how to open your eyes.

That's right. And as long as you hold that image in your imagination, you will not be able to open those eyelids. Because your imagination is where all behavior comes from. First idea, then emotion, then action. That's how it works. Idea, emotion, action. That's right.
You can let that idea sink in now if you like: you can take it in slowly and steadily or you can just "get it." That's right, either way is perfectly perfect for you. That's right.

261

And then you remember to bring your attention to your breathing cycle. Each breathing cycle has two parts, doesn't it? An in-breath and an out-breath. So you can just notice how you breathe: you can begin by breathing in, as if your entire body were a big balloon, and you're filling it with a great big sighing breath, or you can begin by breathing out, out, out, out...to the very last bit of breath, out. Can you not?

And you can take a moment to decide whether you would rather begin on the in-breath or begin on the out breath, it doesn't matter of course. They both take you to the same place: the gateway of hypnotic relaxation; hypnotic trance. Where your focus of attention is drawn inwards, into your inner awareness of your feelings, your thoughts, your memories, where everything pertinent to you is created and experienced. Isn't that right?

It all happens inside, in your inside awareness, the gateway to your subconscious mind where all of your memories, feelings, beliefs, and thoughts are stored. So as you remember how to bring your attention more and more inside, there is a sense of all things outside melting out of your conscious awareness. Just drifting off out of your conscious awareness because you remember how wonderful it feels to be in hypnosis again. And you might wonder, just how deeply down you might go today. And you can wonder, can't you? Of course, it doesn't matter how deeply down you go.

As soon as you close your eyes, and think a thought or imagine an imagining, this process back into hypnosis has already begun. So you can just let it. With each breath you breathe in, you breathe in more relaxation, as muscles loosen and lengthen, becoming soft, and smooth and heavy and even sleepy. That's right. And you can, if you wish, hold that breath for just a moment. Let that wonderful oxygen, Mother Nature's tranquilizer, Mother Nature's pain killer, Mother Nature's own sleepy, drowsy, dozy, drifty drug takes you

262

down. And because you hold it for just a moment, that oxygen, that air, is carried in the blood to each and every cell in your body. And each and every cell in your body soaks up that oxygen like a thirsty sponge, you let go even more, don't you? You can, if you wish.

And why wouldn't you? It is the best feeling in the whole world and so very powerful. Maybe you can't wait to go even deeper, into that place where you learn the best, the fastest, where all imagined behaviors become automatic. That's right. That's how learnings are, aren't they? That's right. So you can let it...if you wish.

And as you breathe out, you release all thoughts of the day...all thoughts that you came in here with and all thoughts of when you leave. Release your attention to those thoughts and bring your attention inwards, to your breathing, to the hearing of my voice and the words that I say, even the pauses and silences between my words, that might take you even deeper down inside.

Going into hypnosis can be like riding along above the waves, drifting up a little and then drifting back down even deeper, that's right, rocking gently, steadily, letting go more and more into that wonderful state of blissful, blessed nothingness where all wonderful new things happen.

And as you go deeper down, deeper down inside your inner awareness, you can begin to think these thoughts.

You are here because you have a dream, a goal you want to accomplish, a way you want to succeed. Only you know what the whole of that is but that is all that is necessary. Think about yourself having accomplished that goal. Look forward for just a moment, will you?

As if you were watching a movie of your future. And suddenly you might find yourself in that movie of your future. You have already accomplished your goal. What does it look like to you? What does it feel like? Are there sounds you can hear? Are there smells you can smell? Can you hear inner choruses of: Atta boy, well done, you did it, didn't you, good for you! You can bask in those inner voices. Perhaps you hear the voices of your greatest supporters, you did it, well done, good for you, way to go, you look great. Tell me how you did it.

Best of all, you can look into the magic mirror of your future...every time I suggest that you look into the magic mirror of your future, you can look and see yourself as you will be, in the weeks or months it will take to get there. See the new, slender, fit you...at the perfect weight for you.

This magic mirror is a 360 degree mirror, so you can see yourself from every angle. Immerse yourself in this vision: you look great! Your clothes look great on you, falling the way you want them to fall, easy, comfortable.

Feel the prideful puffing up of success. Enjoy it. Immerse yourself in it. Take a sensory snapshot of how you look and feel. You can return to that snapshot many times in the next days, weeks and months. Each time you look at that snapshot of you looking into the magic mirror of the future, your motivation will strengthen. You will know without a doubt that you will succeed in reaching this goal. Every time you think about this imagining, your resolve will strengthen. Any doubts or weaknesses or temptations to fall off of your path will dissolve, won't they? The pull towards the future you will be strengthened and renewed.

While you are looking at this sensory snapshot, this imagining that you carry inside, you cannot fail, you cannot weaken, and your motivation will be renewed. You will be pulled back onto this path, because this is the most important happening in your life right now. It is your holy grail. It is the pull of your own needs and desire. Let it pull you towards your goal. Let it carry you. And it will. All you have to do is look at that inner imagining and you will be popped back onto your path, even more strengthened...even more determined.

And, why not? This is what you want. This is why you came to me. This is what you paid your hard-earned money for. This is where you are investing your time and energy. This is the most important thing in your life right now. Life can happen around you and it will but your path will hold you and you will follow that light, won't you? Because this is what you want more than anything else in your life right now. All you have to do is remember how important your goal is.

You are the winner; the rock star, rocking it. This is the state from which you attain all goals. It drives you, carries you, cheers you on. There is a state of mind from which all of us do our best. Think about a time when you were at the top of your game, when you could do no wrong, when you could not fail. It might have been time when things went your way, you had good luck or it might have been a time when you had worked hard to accomplish something and you had really succeeded at something. Think back to a time that you experienced this.

Notice the mind and body sensations. You felt up. You felt energetic, optimistic, happy, powerful, smart, strong, courageous. Maybe there's a sense of a connectedness with Universal or divine energy and you found you could easily draw power from that. Maybe you experience a sense of lightness, powerfulness, courage, or strength. Feel the light. Wrap yourself in the uplifting cocoon of achievement. This state is filled with inner choruses of I can do it, piece of cake, I'm on it, I've got this one, out of my way, coming through. Maybe you feel showered in divine light from which you draw strength, motivation, determination. Maybe you connect to your own inner core of strength and wisdom and draw strength and motivation from that.

This state makes you stand a little taller, shoulders square, foot step secure and determined, jaw set, smile on your face, breathing in success with every breath you take in. Breathing out all doubt, any thoughts of giving up; breathe them away. Yes, of course you can it. Hear yourself say it. Hear my voice say it to you. Hear the voice of the greatest cheerleader in your life. Smell the sweet smell of success. Linger on it. You're on the right path and can stay on it. Eyes front and on the prize: your re-emerged and re-activated perfect eating body, eating only what it needs for perfect fueling.

Every bite we eat is the raw material of every cell that we rebuild, repair, replace. You can build a body made of processed, empty, chemically materials or you can build a clean, strong body of the finest cellular material. It's your choice, isn't it? Your choices, for whatever reasons got you here. It is your choices alone that will create your body of the future.

The body you are building from today forward will find itself drawn to the most nutritious fuel; will taste the wonderful flavors of this perfect fuel, will smell the rich fragrances of the most nutritious fuel. The body that you are building will find less-nutritious foods less compelling, a turnoff really, flat, empty, chemically. You will find that you taste the fake flavors and chemicals and they will turn you off. Your attention will be drawn to the delicious fresh vegetables, perfectly prepared, sweet, delicious fruits, lean but flavorful meats and proteins, whole grains.

The fake processed food will taste like what it is, behind the fake flavor: empty, like cardboard, addicting, compelling but for what? You will suddenly really taste that junk and spit it out.

Your body wisdom will intuitive choose the best fuel. You will eat only enough to be no longer full. You will come to enjoy that feeling of being right on the edge of being hungry. No longer hungry, but not totally stuffed full. You will find that you really love that lean, mean fighting machine feeling as your body takes the good fuel you give it and turn it into pink, new, fresh, strong, healthy cells that become your new, young, energetic, easily moving and active body.

However, whatever, wherever this magically motivational state comes from, whenever you see yourself here, imagine yourself in this state, remember what it feels like to be in this state, any time you create this state with you in the middle of it, anything and everything you set out to do will be charmed. Confidence, courage, motivation, empowerment will flow when in this state. Everything you decide to do is on its way to becoming your new reality.

Science explains this phenomenon but you don't have to understand it to experience it and use it. Put yourself into this state when you visualize the outcome you desire. Put yourself into this state when you start your day. Put yourself into this state when you feel yourself starting to slip back into old ways. Put yourself into this state when you feel doubtful or are wavering or relapsing or falling backwards.

Put yourself into this state and project yourself several months into the future, having achieved your goal. See how you good you look, feel, and sound. See the admiring, respectful, supportive faces of the people who love you; maybe even those who don't.

Whenever you feel yourself weakening or relapsing, turn that channel on and turn it up. Make it bigger and brighter, with lots of vibrant colors. Hear the sounds of success, the atta boys/girls, the "wow, you look great," "how'd you do it?" "what a huge difference!" "way to go!"

This is why you're here. This is why you made that decision to come here. This is why you come to sessions, pay for sessions, do the work you do. This is the most important goal in your life right now. No matter what life throws at you, you can transcend it by keeping your eye on the prize, the gold ring, the end of the rainbow. The good news is that once you've decided to pursue any goal and taken action towards realizing that goal, 75% of your work has already been done.

Anytime you imagine being in this state or feeling in this state, every suggestion that's ever been given will be reinforced. Every time these suggestions are reinforced, you go back into this state from which you cannot fail.

Look into the magic mirror of your future. See the smallest details that puff yourself up with the pride of achievement. Immerse yourself in what you see in the Magic Mirror of Your Future. Feel it. Feel how good it feels to feel slender and fit, at your perfect weight for you. The weight and fitness that makes you smile every time you pass your reflection. The weight and fitness that makes you stand taller and shine from the inside out. Maybe you remember That Girl, as she jumps for joy and throws her hat in the air. That way. That's you!

Look into the magic mirror as you fall asleep. Remind your subconscious mind to do what it does best, while you're sleeping, coming up with all the ways for you to succeed. See yourself in the Magic Mirror every time you look into the mirror; see the you of the future, outlined, coming forward, becoming your reality. You CAN do it. Yes, of course you CAN.

Reverse Metaphor

by Mary Lee LaBay

This technique for accessing information from the subconscious mind is easy to facilitate and elicits intuitive and practical wisdom and information concerning the topic being addressed. It can be used in the following cases:

- When unsure where to start with a client.
- When seeking to discover the most important issue to address, out of a list the client has provided.
- When feeling less than resourceful in choosing the best tool for the presenting issue.
- When the client needs more choices or ideas for resolutions to their issues.
- When searching for the source of chronic illness, pain, and so forth.
- When the client has an issue that they are not comfortable revealing in direct language.
- When there is an extra ten to twenty minutes in your session to fill with productive work.
- When the client is unable to connect with a past life regression, they can start the process through Reverse Metaphor, and the story soon becomes memories of a previous lifetime.

Whether applied in conjunction with an induction or in the middle of the session, here is an example of the language to set up the technique:

"I would like to ask the subconscious mind to create for us a story, a metaphor, which will help us to understand its message.

We may not know where the story begins or ends, or what happens in between, simply allowing it to unfold before us as we proceed through the story.

So if you were telling a story, a fantasy, not a memory, would your story begin indoors or outdoors? And if you were in that scene, what would you be doing?"

Once they begin to tell the story, simply continue to ask them, *"And what happens next?"* Write their responses in a column.

When the story is complete, go back over the details of the story, individually and starting from the top, asking the client how that relates to their life here.

For example: *"You mentioned that you were walking along a dirt path. If that path was symbolic of something in your life here, what would that mean? You mentioned that there were trees on the right side of the path. What would those trees represent in your own life?"* And so forth...

Bear in mind that if the client begins to tell you a memory or experience from this life, gently guide them back to a fantasy story. While the memory may also have a connection to the presenting problem, and can also be addressed, the object of this exercise is to allow the subconscious mind to communicate without interference from the conscious mind. It is very closely related to dream interpretation, which can also be facilitated through the use of a modified version of this technique.

The Ceramic Vase

by Katherine Zimmerman

Rebuilding Self-esteem

Following induction and deepener....

One day, when she was out taking a walk, a young woman came across a very old ceramic vase. She could see that it had been beautiful when it was new. The colors, although faded, were still formed into various shapes and pictures. And the shape of the vase was quite striking.

But the vase had been out in the elements, battered by rain and wind. Over time chips had broken off and there were small cracks in the sides. The handle was broken. It was obvious to the woman that it would no longer hold water or be an attractive addition to her garden.

But maybe, just maybe she could repair this vase. It would be a wonderful gift for her dear friend. Her friend had been on an extended trip and she wanted to surprise her with this gift when she returned.

She picked up the vase and carried it home that very day. She placed the vase in the greenhouse in back of her home. And there it sat for many days and weeks while the woman thought about how to correctly apply the repairs.

After much thought she went to the pottery shop in town and took a class on making pottery. She learned everything that she needed to know about paint, and clay and the proper material to seal the vase. She wanted to do a really good job so she paid close attention in class. She learned all about glazes and types of clay. She learned how to make a ceramic vase from beginning to end. She took her time and made several ceramic items. She started with something simple. First a simple plate, next she tackled a cup and then a small vase. Each project looked better than the last one.

When she took her final class project out of the kiln she felt confident and she knew that now she was ready to repair the beautiful vase that she'd found. In class she'd learned that repairing a vase was quite different from making one from start to finish. But she knew that she could call on her teacher from class to guide her in repairing this beautiful vase.

And so she began. She took her time with the repairs. Each day she would mend or re-mold a small section. Then she would stand back and admire her work. Yes, it was coming along nicely. And with each small change, her confidence grew.

Slowly, gently she filled in the cracks. She added clay to the handle and reshaped it. She filled in the chips. Then, after much love and attention and some skillful work, the vase was ready to be repainted. She returned to the pottery shop and carefully picked out just the right colors to decorate the vase and restore the original picture.

She waited until the light in the greenhouse was bright so that she could easily see where to apply the new paint. With a gentle stroke, she began repainting the once beautiful vase. Each day she worked diligently on a small section of the picture. When the light changed, she stepped back and waited for another day. She was positive that if she just took her time she could restore this vase to its former beauty.

Finally, the vase was done. She was sure that it was as beautiful as it had ever been. She was proud of herself for her accomplishment. In all the time that she had worked on this vase she had never looked at the bottom. Imagine her delight when she turned the vase over and discovered a positive, inspirational message carved into the clay. The words were still clear and easy to read. She read the words, closed her eyes and let them sink in.

(Pause)

And, at last, she was ready to place the vase in the garden where her friend could enjoy it upon her return. She was excited to have finished the vase because she had a strong feeling that her friend would be back very soon. She walked all around the garden that day, looking for the perfect place for the vase. And there it was...next to the bench and under an enormous shade tree. Her favorite flowers grew all around the tree. It was the perfect place to show off her vase and still keep it protected. She placed the vase on a small, sturdy stand, filled it with potting soil and planted her favorite plant. When she was finished, she sat on the bench and admired her work.

When her friend returned the woman could see the excitement on her face when she saw the gift. And she was very pleased. All her hard work and patience had paid off.

Cleaning out the Rooms

by Toni Macri-Reiner

Following Induction:

I use some sort of deepener that lets them move downward such as through a building. This is an example, as any sort of going down deepener will work.

Now that you are so comfortably relaxed, feeling safe...Begin imagining yourself drifting down through a busy office building at the end of a long day...each floor becoming quiet...as the lights dim for the night..The top floor quieting as all the high powered executives begin their transition from work mode to relaxing and letting go...The workers on each floor below leave for home and as a hush falls over the work space...the energy of the day...just...floats...away. That's right...the quiet deepens as you descend... imagining the look of the building as the power systems...turn off, allowing the release of energy...becoming quieter & more peaceful with each floor you descend.

You just observe the process of slowing down...noticing the lobby...the last of the workers saying goodnight...letting yourself drift even further down...

You find yourself at the end of a long corridor, the hush settling around you like a comfortable blanket...you instinctively know that...you are alone in this place... safe...secure... enjoying the beauty of this hidden level where your imagination becomes even more powerful...And you notice this corridor curving off in the distance, making it impossible to see where it actually goes...now noticing...the beautiful doors recessed into each side of the hallway stretching...all along the walls...

And each door is labeled in bold lettering...The first door is labeled _____ *(whatever issue they have mentioned. I might use "weight" or a person, ex husband, an emotion, etc...)*

Feel the weight of the door shift and open slightly as you turn the knob...you reach your hand into the room, flip on the light switch...Now, make your way across this dusty room...full of things...ideas...beliefs...which are no longer needed...Unrecognizable piles...Finding the window...pull back the drapes and feel the sunlight flowing in from this large window...Open the window and enjoy the warm, gentle breeze that floats in, carrying the gentlest whisper of....fresh spring days...As you look back to the room... notice...cleaning supplies in the corner...and begin sweeping, dusting, sorting and even throwing out those old outdated beliefs and thoughts you have needlessly kept stored.

I'll be quiet now as you do what your unconscious mind feels is necessary to freshen this room of _____. And when it feels clean and updated, just nod your head....

Depending on the client I might suggest other rooms to visit. (I once suggested a room where a family of germs lived. I pointed out how badly the parents were trying to provide for their small germ children. The germs just wanted to go about their business. They were the good germs; they helped people build up resistance, etc...)

After one or two rooms, I tell them I will be quiet as they move down the hallway as far as they'd like to go...cleaning opening windows...refreshing; not really needing to look too closely as most of what the rooms contain are unrecognizable now...old crumbling stuff stored from long ago & just taking up space.

They are asked to nod or lift a finger when finished.

This place may be accessed anytime you relax yourself .....

This is more of an outline than an exact script. I vary it from client to client. Many clients have expressed how much better they feel after having "cleaned".

Fade to Black

by Sherry Hood

This is a multi-purpose script designed to be used for many different problems. It is important to know which areas a client wishes to release and which areas a client wishes to expand upon before beginning this session.

I have left blank spaces "_____" throughout the script. Problems such as shame, guilt, fear etc could fill the blank areas. Further down into the script, there are opportunities to fill the blank spaces with positive qualities one might wish to increase; i.e. confidence, self esteem, honoring self, etc.

We are about to release some residual elements that have been affecting your Conscious waking state as well as your dream time.

Picture or imagine a bank of monitors that are in front of you. Each monitor represents different aspects of your life. Some of these aspects are things that you might like to keep close, increase or bring forward into your life and there are some aspects that are represented on these monitors that are ready to be released from your life. You can choose to fade them to black and release them completely.

As you visualize or imagine these monitors, notice that each one has a label at the bottom of the screen. On the screen, the area of your life that is represented is playing, just like a movie.

This information could also come to you through your

auditory senses or possibly a feeling, a thought or an awareness.

The first monitor is labeled _____. See, feel or become aware of the different aspects of that experience being played out. The negative aspects of this event have been troubling you and getting in the way of your current life situation. It is time to eliminate these difficult aspects from your life.

I would like you to take a nice, cleansing breath and as you exhale, allow any body tension to dissipate. Now, imagine or visualize turning the dial on the _____ monitor and fade it to black. As the images on the monitor move out of focus and dim, and then fade to black, you are releasing past negative events surrounding the _____ experience. Allow yourself to experience the emotions and feelings that go with taking control of this area of your life.

There is a second monitor that needs your attention today. This monitor is labeled _____. From our conversation, it is clear that you have been very hard on yourself about this. You have learned and grown from this experience and it is time to move forward and leave the past, in the past, where it belongs. Go ahead and begin turning the dial down. Watch the picture become blurry and unfocused and then finally, fade to black. And as the monitor goes black, the trauma of this past experience also fades away. It fades from your thoughts, your feelings and your life. This does not mean that the memories around this experience go away. This simply means that the symptoms and problems that have been affecting you no longer dominate your daily life. You can become free to move in a new direction.

As you release these troubling aspects from your past, you are clearing the way for an entirely new future...a future that is filled with joy and happiness.

Notice the monitor that is labeled _____. _____has played an enormous role in your life. You have taken it on and made it your own. As you look at this now, you may be able to see that _____is a debilitating problem. It is like looking at a life through a dirty window. Take hold of that dial on the _____ monitor and fade it to black.

Allow yourself to experience the emotions and feelings of letting _____ go. In the past, these feelings and symptoms were invited guests but you always reserve the right to change your mind. You are now telling these long staying guests that it is time to leave. They have no choice but to leave because you are in charge. You are the one that gets to decide and you now decide to live a life of clarity, peace and purpose.

I would like you to take a look at the next monitor. This monitor is labeled _____. Even the word, _____, is heavy and harsh. _____ has kept you from achieving your goals. It has stood in your way at every turn. _____ has affected your health physically, emotionally and mentally. Turn the dial on the _____ monitor all the way down and fade it to black.

As you make these positive changes in your life, you become clear. You are easily able to see how these issues clouded your life and held you in place. You are connecting the dots and this is empowering for you. Imagine or visualize that you are removing a heavy cloak of burden that you have been wearing for a long time. Allow yourself to experience how much lighter you feel without this heavy weight.

There is a monitor in front of you that is labeled _____. You know that it is tied to fear. You have been afraid to make decisions. Decisions have caused you to experience feelings of _____ and insecurity. Turn that dial on the _____ monitor all the way down and fade it to black. As you fade the _____ monitor to black, let yourself experience feelings of freedom, safety and security. Your thoughts are more precise, even your memory is improving.

There is a rather large monitor that is labeled _____. _____ has been such a culprit for you. It has attached itself to every area of your life. It has made itself quite comfortable and at home within your life. You know that you can make the choice to overpower _____ at anytime. You may even decide to banish _____ from your life once and for all. If you are ready, turn that _____ dial all the way down and fade it to black. Feel yourself becoming even more empowered.

Notice the monitor that is labeled _____. This monitor is also tied to fear and insecurity. You are taking your power back now. I want you to give yourself permission to be strong. Within your mind now, I want you to say, "I give myself permission to be empowered". As you say it, you bring it forth into your life. You are expecting a good life, and so it is. Fade the _____ monitor to black and release that _____ feeling from your life entirely.

And now you can go to work, increasing the positive aspects of your life and bringing them into the forefront.

Notice now that the _____ monitor is black. You can turn it up, bringing light and clarity to that monitor. Turn it all the way up now and as you turn it up, allow yourself to experience the positive feelings that go with that. As you turn the _____ monitor all the way up, so too, you are turning up your _____ abilities. You are turning up the calm, relaxed feelings that go with _____.

Notice the _____ monitor is also black. Turn it up as far as it goes. All the way up and watch as the screen lights up completely. You are fine tuning all of your excellent qualities and releasing those which no longer serve you well. You are inviting excellent qualities to increase and expand as you dismiss things that no longer fit into your life.

There is a monitor that is labeled _____. I think that it is time to turn that monitor on. Once it is on, turn that dial as far as it will go, all the way up. It is time to honor the person that you are. It is time to allow all of your beauty to shine out for everyone to see. It is time to start living your life fully, accepting all of the warmth and joy in life while letting go of negativity. Old patterns are broken and new healthy patterns are established.

Script for Premature Ejaculation (PE)

by Stephanie Conkle

This is quick and easy! Do whatever induction method you would like...in this case, quicker is better...haha! Pun intended!

Be sure to *emphasize* the *italicized words* and <u>really *verbally* punch and pause on the underlined words (they are direct suggestions)</u>...

I know a guy who was deceived by the media and random street talk. He is a friend of mine and I have cared about him for a *very long, long, long* time now. He was fooled into thinking that men should keep an erection for a *very long time*, how those fake men in pornos have been trained to do, instead of realizing <u>now</u>, and <u>believing</u> the truth, which in fact, is that the average length of time for an erection is only 5-7 minutes long. And <u>you are</u> more than likely to go the full 7 minutes or more, but any time *much, much longer* than that could even indicate a sign of a medical problem, like the other guy I knew who had an erection four hours long and his wife (*or lover, girlfriend, partner, etc.*) had to take him to see a doctor.

So he thought the thing to do is not to think about it at all and be <u>satisfied</u> in the moment <u>by</u> giving and receiving pleasure freely, by adding more foreplay and <u>making her come</u> to understand how much he loved her by *taking the time* to work on her needs <u>first</u>, knowing somewhere deep down that the more thought he put into her, the *longer he could get off* of putting the pressure all on himself, and now

283

he could confidently ejaculate in a timely matter, when it was *just right* for both of them, not even thinking about it, by allowing his intuition to take over, <u>and</u> realizing that <u>holding a longer erection</u> mattered less than the quality of pleasure he gave his lover in all sorts of creative <u>and</u> fun ways they loved, <u>clinching</u> their affection for each other, and experiencing better orgasms. Now <u>when</u> he wants, he can have sex freely, and whenever they <u>need it</u> to *last a while longer*, he remembers to *spend more time on her*.

In a moment I am going to slowly count up to ten and you will go 10 times, 10...times, 10...times deeper and deeper in trance. 1-2-3-4-5-6-7-8-9-10.

Using your imagination, go inside yourself and find the factory that controls your sexual activity. Look around and find the control dials. One dial controls penis firmness, one controls penis size, etc., and one controls the length of time to ejaculation. Find that dial. Now notice there is a countdown clock associated with that dial that gets triggered upon penetration and masturbation. Observe how many minutes are on the screen of the clock. Move the dial back and forth and notice the minutes going up and down. Good!

Now, move those dials until they are set to the minimum time you would like to hold onto an erection. Next to that is a dial for which you can set the maximum time you care to have an erection last. Go ahead and set that time. Good. Now observe all the other dials and confidently make any adjustments or tweaks necessary. Excellent!

Now take one more look to be sure you are completely satisfied with the adjustments you just made, and when you are certain, find the big red button on the wall and push it to lock in the settings. Indicate to me when you have locked in those settings by nodding your head or lifting your finger...

(*Wait for response. Please do not rush it.*)

Fantastic! Are you sure you have them set in and don't want to change them? Here is your last chance to make tweaks. Excellent!

(*Either emerge him now or count him down again and give more metaphors that deal with the pleasure of taking time to do things, like eating a gourmet meal, drinking a fine wine, relaxing in a warm bath, etc.*)

White Canvas

by Jodie Tessier

Release Work in Somnambulism

A door now appears in front of you and you know that once you pass through that doorway and experience what is there, you will be better than ever before. You reach for the door handle and with the greatest of ease, because you know you are ready for change and resolution, you open the door.

You step into a large white room, so white, it takes your eyes a moment to adjust to the vibrant white surfaces...a white ceiling and floor...white walls. You become aware of yourself now and you may be nude as a newborn or wearing all white clothing...either way, you are completely comfortable and at ease. White is a symbol of purity and new beginnings. Every canvas starts off white before there is art made on it. Being nude or in white clothing represents your subconscious mind and self at the time of your birth. As an infant you were a white canvas, pure and suggestible to all positive and negative conditioning.

Standing there in all of your purity, you feel the weight of something in your hand. It is the weight of a large, permanent black marker. This marker, for the time being, represents all negative conditioning and thoughts that you feel have been imposed on you throughout your life...imposed on you by others or yourself.

So now, holding this permanent marker, I want you to walk to one of the clean white walls and begin to write, with the marker, words that represent all of the negative conditionings and thoughts within you. The more impact these negative conditionings or thoughts have had on your life, the larger the words can be written. If and when you run out of writing space on that wall you may move to the other three walls, the ceiling and the floor. You are able to write on any surface in the room. Take this time now in the privacy of your subconscious to write all those negative conditionings and thoughts. And when you feel you are complete, please indicate to me by nodding your head.

(*Once client has nodded their head*)

Wonderful. Now that the white surfaces of the room are scribed with all those negative conditionings and thoughts I would like you to take the permanent black marker and start to write on your nude body or white clothing all the negative thoughts or feelings you've ever had towards or imposed upon yourself. Write words to represent all the negative thoughts and feelings you've ever had towards yourself over your body. Once again, take the time to write on every available surface of your nude body or white clothing until you feel you are done. Please indicate to me when you are complete.

(*Once client has nodded their head again*)

Take this time to look around the white room now scribed with permanent black marker and take the time to look at your body or clothing full of negative thoughts and feelings. You can almost feel the weight of each mark, of each word as it bears down on you and your surroundings. Everywhere you look there are negative things scribed, all around you, this makes it so difficult to think of anything else.

Now, think to yourself how wonderful it would be to be rid of all these negative words and thoughts. How wonderful it would be to be a white canvas once again. But those words have been scribed in permanent marker, they cannot be washed away. Here is where the beauty and the power of your mind become so handy and so helpful:

Standing in the middle of your heavily scribed room you suddenly feel one drop of water spill onto your cheek. You know it came from somewhere above you...but you're not sure where. You can feel the cool, refreshing sensation as the water drop caresses down your face and drops to the floor.

Instinctively you bring your hand up to your now wet cheek and when you pull your hand back to examine it, you notice it is covered in black smudges. You think, "How is this possible? All of those negative thoughts were scribed permanently, never to be washed away or changed..." Ah, but you have the power to rewrite and recreate your belief system. You can feel that power above you now...in the form of a soft rainstorm manifesting itself in the very room you stand in. You are not alarmed or frightened, in fact, you anticipate the cleansing of your mind.

Drop after drop of water spills down from the ceiling now, faster and faster...more and more rain drops are spilling and splashing on every surface. You feel the water hitting every part of your body. You hear the rain splattering on the floor and walls. And with each raindrop you feel the cleansing of all those negative issues. Every negative belief, thought, conditioning that has ever been imposed on you by others or by your own self is being washed away gently and thoroughly. The water collecting on the floor is darkened gray but it is draining somewhere so you don't have to stand in the residue of all that negativity. As you are cleansed and the surfaces in the room are washed clean you feel an overwhelming sense of relief and comfort. You are anticipating being able to look around the room and at yourself and see nothing but white, clean, pure and ready.

Nod to me to indicate when you and your room's surfaces have been cleansed with the rain and are free of all those negative conditions and thoughts that you were so sure were permanent.

(*Once the client has nodded their head*)

Amazing work. Take this moment to relish your success. Take a look around the room and at the proof of the power of your subconscious mind. There is a mirror on one of the walls in front of you. Take pride in looking at yourself and seeing that you are now a white canvas once again, ready to be recreated with new and positive art. What wonderful power you have demonstrated over your once "thought-to-be-permanent" issues. They didn't stand a chance against your cleansing rain and power.

You are now feeling so much relief and confidence in yourself and your future. Once again you feel the weight of something in your hand. This time the weight is that of a paintbrush. This is no ordinary paintbrush. It has the capability to paint any color you can think of, any color that exists in the universe. Your subconscious mind has no limits of the beauty it can create with this paintbrush. You and your mind are a white canvas. It is time to take that paintbrush and paint positive thoughts and suggestions to yourself over all the surfaces of the room and on yourself.

Paint words, symbols and pictures to represent positive

thoughts and suggestions that you now want as part of your life and subconscious mind. If you paint it, it will be so. You have the power to recreate your belief system and be the artist of your own life. Paint with all the colors of the universe, paint positive thoughts and suggestions about you, your life and your future. Paint all the positive things you want to incorporate within yourself and it will be so.

When you have completed your masterpiece of positive thoughts and suggestions, take a moment to appreciate all your hard work and beauty. At any time in the future you can simply remember and revisit this room of positive thoughts and suggestions. And when you visit in your subconscious mind you experience this wonderful feeling every time. You can feel the power of this room at any time in the future when you simply visit here in the quiet of your mind.

And each and every time you visit this beautiful room of your art you find it easier and easier to find and feel the power of the positive thoughts and suggestions you have created...easier and easier to find and feel the power of the positive thoughts and suggestions you have painted for yourself here.

Bridge of Light - Activating Your Multi-Dimensional Light Body

by Sally Homes Reed

We all know that Hypnosis is a wonderful, versatile tool that supports positive change in many ways, including what is beginning to be called Spiritual Hypnosis. Hypnosis allows us to access all levels of consciousness. Working in a light trance will enhance your spiritual, metaphysical and mystical practice. Remember, this is about your empowerment, so don't be surprised when you begin to see yourself in a whole new light.

Allow yourself to continue to experience this deep state of relaxation...becoming more and more comfortable...as your mind becomes calmer and clearer...with every breath you take...and with each word I speak...simply letting go of any attachments to anyone or anything...allowing everything unimportant to simply fade away and disappear completely...

And now...with every breath you take...breathing in all that you need...breathe out any negative memories, thoughts or feelings...any doubt or worry or fear... breathing out anything you may have been carrying before now...any shame or blame or pain...no longer afraid to step out of your old comfort zone...

As you begin to reach for the stars...letting go of

grasping or resistance...simply letting go completely with each exhale...really relaxing into the emptiness...and as you do...choose to let go of everybody and everything...letting go of all energies you may have been carrying before now...release all thoughts and opinions... forgive yourself for whatever you may have done to create or contribute to any problems...past, present and future...becoming more and more flexible...resting in awareness...because THIS changes THAT...

As you look to the stars...beginning to harmonize with the new frequencies that are coming to you now...causing a wave of reorganization on all levels of consciousness...naturally adjusting to what is most comfortable for you...as you allow yourself to enter your imagination...into your own mind's eye...to that part of you already floating in and out of this place where you can feel more comfortable than you have ever felt before...creating this new space within for you to begin to receive whatever it is you are wanting to receive...starting right now...

Letting your Higher consciousness simply take over...because your Higher consciousness knows exactly what to do and is doing it right now...in just the right way...taking all the time you need...as you simply continue to relax completely...becoming more and more comfortable...with every breath you take... breathing in love and appreciation and gratitude...

And as you continue...inhaling slowly and deeply...letting your body expand... filling yourself completely...what if you can begin to imagine opening up every cell of your body...and...releasing... releasing...releasing...whatever needs to be released ...on all levels of consciousness...

Breathing in...all the way up to your collar bone...once again...holding for just a moment...as you trigger the relaxation response in the center of your brain... letting this fresh oxygen wash through every cell of your body...from the top of your head...to the tips of your fingers...to the soles of your feet...

And as you exhale...simply open your mind...release your thoughts...and connect with your heart... **continue to tune into your body more and more efficiently**...because now your inner mind will continue working all by itself to open you up to the truth within...allowing you to change your way of life at the core...letting your true self shine through...

Allowing you to feel better in every way...breathe in unconditional love and life... breathe out any disbelief, fear, tension, holding or resistance...release all obstacles...simply letting go completely of whatever is preventing you from reaching your dreams...with every breath you take...becoming more and more comfortable with the process of change...because change always happens... allowing you to accept the flow of change in an easy and effortless way...starting right NOW...

And as you do...allowing your Higher consciousness to simply take over...because your Higher consciousness knows exactly what to do and is doing right now in just the right way...taking all the time you need...allowing it to happen automatically without having to think about it...as you easily and effortlessly ...release the past...reset those old dysfunctional default settings...and step into your new future that supports you completely...

And it all begins with the breath...new life always begins with that first breath of awareness...

So from now on...today and every day as you step into your new future that is light and joyful...whenever you feel any stress in your life...any of the doubt or worry or fear that you used to have before now...any untrue, critical, or judgmental thoughts...any anxieties...or anything you may feel uncertain about before now...or anything that is holding you back from having a life that is better than you ever imagined...

Then...you will simply stop...bring your full awareness into the present moment... and take a nice deep breath into your heart...into the center of yourself... into what you may begin to imagine as your Core*Star...as you begin to breathe in all the love and goodness you need ...

Breathing in love and appreciation and gratitude into every cell of your body... right into the heart of your own DNA...releasing...releasing...releasing...all that does not support you completely in making these positive changes in your life... starting right now...

Allowing this wonderful sense of well-being to wash through every cell of your body...filling you with compassion and insight...from the top of your head...to the tips of your fingers...to the soles of your feet...restoring all to balance and harmony...on all levels of consciousness...and just let that continue automatically so you don't have to think about it...

Now...let's send your awareness down to the soles of your feet for just a moment...what if you can imagine that you discover you seem to have magnets on the soles of your feet that can connect you into the Earth's magnetic crystalline grid...perhaps **feeling fully grounded and supported by the Earth below you**...allowing your energy to be renewed by this connection...

Now send your awareness deep into the center of the Earth, grounding into the crystalline energy core of what you may begin to imagine as the Earth*Star... here... begin to deeply draw all the energy you discover there...this crystalline light Earth Core energy...feel it travelling back up...entering through the soles of your feet...easily moving up through your legs...through your lower back...and travelling up...and opening...and activating all of your energy centers...

Spinning your new life into motion...right to left...in tune with the rhythm of the Earth...and just like the Earth revolves around the Sun...and our solar system revolves around the Galactic Core...continue to let this energy spiral up through your entire belly...your solar plexus...through your heart...up through your throat...through the base of your neck...into all parts of your brain...filling your whole head completely...front, back, and center ...

Now take a moment to imagine every cell of your body completely filled with this crystalline light Earth energy...opening easily and effortlessly to receive...on all levels of consciousness...and let that continue in whatever way works best for you and your whole body...that's right...

Now send your awareness to the top of your head for just a moment...and what if you can imagine that you can expand your consciousness out through the top of your head...up through all 12 dimensions...spiraling up...moving out of space and time...leaving the old behind...and stepping through the portal into this expanded consciousness...as if the Universe has opened its doors for you...allowing you to uplift the frequency of your vibration...letting in more and more light...and as you move through the gateway to all understanding...emerging as you do...shifting your reality...stepping into the light of new possibilities...

And before you appears a shining, shimmering, brilliant BRIDGE OF LIGHT...as you step over...allow your Divine Self to guide you into your highest and best multi-dimensional Self...activating your Light Body...bringing it alive inside you... and forever be changed...activating all the transformation that is now occurring on all levels of consciousness...and all that you know that means...

Simply continue breathing easily and effortlessly as you imagine the feeling of this activation of your Light Body surrounding you completely...seeing yourself as a beautiful Soul...sparking a greater facet of who you are...where you connect with what you may begin to imagine as your Soul*Star...your Divinity...your celestial Home...your own Soul frequency.. your Soul Truth...your "I AM" Presence...

Here discovering your deepest values and your highest purpose...envisioning your ideal future waiting for you there...in total comfort and ease...enjoying the flow of life...aligning with what makes you happy...discovering what you want and need for your own well-being...feeling all your emotions to completion...embracing it all with graceful acceptance...and dissolving anything that may have been in the way of creating a life that is better than you ever imagined...

Feel what is real and right...connecting with your own inner guidance...resonating with your highest good... recovering the full dimensionality of your Being...becoming a wholly conscious creator...with every step you take...reaching higher and higher...

Until you discover a beautiful golden white crystalline light...filled with all the colors of the rainbow...brighter than all the light you have yet encountered...a pulsing radiance...showering down from the Quantum Field of ALL THAT IS... what you may begin to imagine you can call the All*Star...where All is Light... divine radiance...the Great Central Sun...at the center of the Universe...humming with the sacred elemental sound of Om...

Stepping into this light from Source...blending in...merging...into what seems like shimmering golden liquid light...dissolving away any heaviness...any density...any attempts to control...any old programming...any imprints or blocks...any attachment to cause and effect...any old survival consciousness...any opposing force...allowing anything that does not support you to simply dissolve away and disappear completely...restoring all to balance, harmony and perfection...

With a knowing that NOW...you are in the Universe...and the Universe is in you... in tune with the energy of creation...evolving new magical ways of being...

 Now imagine following these beautiful luminous golden rays that are showering back down...travelling on this beam of light all the way back to here...allowing your Light Body to begin surrounding you completely with its presence...sealing yourself in...feeling safe and secure in the stillness in the center of yourself... embodying this new light...radiating this full spectrum of unconditional love, and light, and life...feeling a greater influence...a greater presence...a greater personal sovereignty...

With all the courage you need to support you completely as you begin to create your own unique path.. bringing to light previously unrealized talents and gifts... connecting to your own intuition...merging with all aspects of the mystery of your true self...fully integrating all facets of your Beingness...coming into unity and completeness...in all layers, levels, and dimensions...throughout all time and space and realities...

Discovering new insights and creative solutions...with your new and powerful feelings of comfort, confidence, and wellbeing...fully present in your body... being thoroughly grounded and supported by the Earth below you...holding the promise of new life...allowing it all to unfold easily and effortlessly...in a whole new way...as you begin to have a more powerful relationship to life...and all that you know that means...

Now, imagine all the love and goodness you need filling you completely...from the top of your head...to the tips of your fingers...to the soles of your feet...and then expanding out into your entire life...restoring a state of grace...in balance and harmony...creating emotional wellness...realizing the power of your full presence and awareness...right now...bringing success to all areas of your life...feel like you have it NOW...because you can, and you will, and you do...allow it to happen automatically...and begin to notice what is different...starting right NOW...

As you begin to enjoy the experience...as the inner work continues...now...as you begin to shift over to a wonderful, refreshed, alert waking state...letting all the benefits expand...as you begin to notice very pleasant changes taking place in your life...starting right NOW!

So in just a moment...or whenever you chose to...bring your focus and attention back to your full awakening awareness...return to the safe and reassuring state of being fully connected to your Light Body...your Highest and Best Self...your Soul Truth...your sense of personal power...your extraordinarily capable mind...your power to choose...fully present in each moment...

Words of Flight

by Alina Robinson

Release limiting thoughts and feelings with this guided imagery...

Imagine yourself walking into a large green open field. Soft sloping hills surround you in every direction. Feel the gentle breeze through your hair, the warmth of the midday sun shining down on your skin.

Up ahead in the distance you see a very large, colorful balloon against the blueness of the afternoon sky. As you start to walk towards it you stop for a moment to listen to the beautiful sounds of the birds chirping with happiness...listen to the beautiful sound.

Continue walking towards the balloon...notice there is a large basket attached to the bottom of it. You now realize that this is a colorful hot air balloon high above your head. You stop to just take in the vast greatness of it...the beautiful vibrant colors of blue...green...red...yellow... and orange that glow in the sunshine.

Step into the basket...good...and take a look in the basket you see several packages wrapped in brown paper...Each is a different size. Take a closer look and you can see each one has a label. These labels are all of your negative thoughts and feelings...all of those feelings that no longer serve you any purpose.

Today, your purpose is to release all of these thoughts and feelings and feel the freedom that comes from doing that...so reach down now and untie the ropes that hold you to the ground and start to feel yourself drifting and floating...drifting and floating...up into the afternoon sky. The gentle breeze is blowing through your hair...the sun is warm on your face...you are drifting and floating.

I want you to pick up one of the packages that are traveling with you and take notice of the label and...as you become aware of what negative thought or feeling you are holding...allow yourself to now just throw it out of the balloon. And as you do this, feel the balloon float a little higher into the sky.

Now take the next package, noticing the negative thought or feeling, and toss it out of the basket...feeling yourself, drifting and floating...higher.

As you take each package and toss it over the side of the basket...you can feel how much higher and faster you go in the balloon. How light you are feeling...drifting and floating...lighter and lighter...faster and faster.

Now allow yourself to just take a moment and throw out any remaining packages of negative thoughts and feelings that might be left with you...excellent...feeling how much lighter you feel. With this new sense of lightness you are feeling fantastic...such freedom from all of the negativity that was holding you down, holding you back.

Now just allow yourself to enjoy this feeling, and as you do this, I want you to also take notice of yourself...take a bit of time and see the beauty of you. Appreciate how positive and beautiful you are...so beautiful...so free...so positive.

As the hot air balloon begins to descend down to the earth,

notice that you still feel light and free. What a great feeling! Allow yourself to step out of the basket of the balloon and plant your feet on the ground...feel the energy that Mother Earth sends through your feet all the way to the top of your head. This is a gift from Mother Earth...sent to fill you up where all that negative used to be...a gift of love especially for you.

The Shift - Mind and Body

by Donna Carter

Before you take on any exercise routine be sure you have checked with your physician. You can add any induction and deepener to the beginning of this and you can add your own count out at the end.

Italics: soften voice. Capitals: enhance voice. In parenthesis is just for you.

Changing your perspective...changes your view. You know this to be true... because if you are looking at something and then take a step to the right or left... your view of it changes. Just as...if you know something and then learn something new, your view...will change.

For example, let us imagine for a moment...you are on a river island...a river like the Yellowstone River. A river SO big...that it can fork around a piece of land... creating an island so big, it has houses and roads, trees and bushes...where deer like to live and hide...and the only way you can see the other side is to walk around to it. This...is an island...a big island. One that is surrounded by the river and you want to cross the river to get to the mainland. In order to do so....from one perspective...the water is rushing... the width too wide...you would definitely get wet and depending on the depth and swiftness of the water it could become dangerous.

As you stand there, on the river bank, lean over and grab some pebbles in your hand.

303

Standing on the riverbank...you might even think...there is no way to move across. However, once you take a step forward...Yes! (say this with Laughter and Joy) you TAKE A STEP FORWARD, walking the beach...

Taking a moment as you walk to imagine and allow any frustrations, sorrows, anything that is no longer needed...It's time to move forward...and attach these old burdens to the pebbles in your hand.

...The scenery is changing as you continue to move forward...you...start noticing positive things you've never noticed before...

Starting now, more and more, you will be able to shift your thoughts and the way you think about situations...to find solutions...to find the positives in the world around you. For example: Have you ever seen someone win something they have worked hard for? Where they cross the finish line and punch the sky? (Get excited when you say this) ...so excited...so proud!

Just for a moment, pretend YOU ARE that person, right now...imagine it...be there...feel it...hear the sounds...smell the smells...It IS...you...just finished walking a 5 k or if your real energetic, running a half marathon...and you cross the finish line...YES!!! It is SO exciting. Exhilarating! And this feeling...this accomplishment has you looking for the next time you can feel that successful feeling...mmm...it feels good...doesn't it...to...walk toward a goal...to...work toward solutions. Be that person for a second...take a deep breath in...and let it out... ahh...accomplishment.

Take another moment and imagine you turn to someone you know...and you tell them "I want this! I know my goal! To seek health and the information that will lead me to it."

Just saying it out loud...hardens your resolve. You know...what you want...a healthy mind and body.

You are able to shift your thoughts to the positive and look at the positive aspects of living...enjoying every day. You become more and more aware that you want to be active...so active...and this activity has you looking into how you can gain better health in all areas of your life...exercise, nutrition and the nutrients your body seeks.

You will become more and more aware that you can find the information you need, with strength and determination. Those solutions...are right at your fingertips... Starting today...you find solutions. You change your view until the answers you seek are right in front of you.

EXERCISING your understanding that YOU CAN pay attention to your environment in a new and improved way...You know life is about the journey and ...so is moving forward...walking forward. Seeking ways to move forward... faster ...and with more skill...

This journey has you saying to yourself, "I love to move my body. I know my body will respond to my goals because I am so comfortable and at ease and going at my own pace."

It doesn't matter whether you're walking or running...it's about finding what your body needs, seeking those solutions...Saying to yourself, "I always feel relaxed and happy when I begin my exercise for the day. Exercise makes me happy and energized. I feel relaxed, mentally alert, and better able to carry on with my day."

YOU CAN imagine it...six months from now...how healthy you look...fresh and ready for your day...see it. Feel it. So excited....Energized from the power within that allows you to know you have SO many ways to create your own positives in the world around you. And each time you visualize this scenario...it gets clearer and clearer. Because you get closer to it each and every time you practice moving forward.

...And you realize, as you walk along the island river bank...moving forward, step by step...just now coming into view...is a bridge...and you have made a profound discovery! Solutions are in the process of moving forward...seeking answers... Seeking those bridges...inside of each and every one of us...We are much more than we think we are.

Not only did this movement forward help you cross a river without getting your feet wet, avoiding potential dangers...it has also allowed you to realize...that changing your perception...changes the rules, it changes the way you think ...forever. Which is a good thing...to move forward, to make progress...and to realize that there are answers...inside you... strengths, resourcefulness, skills, abilities...yours...when you need them.

Knowing...you can continue to seek solutions and move forward in a productive way...by simply taking a nice deep breath in and letting it out...Relaxing and learning.

Now every time you practice hypnosis, either by listening to the sound of my voice or by purposefully sitting down and taking a nice deep breath in and then letting it out...you increase your self-satisfaction, increase your confidence... relaxing...remembering...how life changes...by changing your perception.

Simply now visualize, imagine or pretend, that you are lying down on your bed at the end of the day...knowing that each and every day...when you lay down to sleep...you allow yourself to drift completely and comfortably into sleep, sleeping soundly, so that any of these old frustrations, sorrows, anything that is no longer of use to you...can simply be let go...so those old, exhausted burdens become like the pebbles, that you once held in your hand so long ago...

Take a moment to imagine...tossing those pebbles back into the river, as you cross that bridge. You can imagine what that would be like, if you toss the pebbles right back out into the river, washed away...so easily cleansed...the weight has been lifted, you are light... free.... ready to make progress...more cleansed, more renewed, strengthened, focused and calm... each and every day, each and every way, getting better and better...those old thoughts and ideas just become so silly when you realize how strong you are. And as you grow stronger and stronger, you realize more and more that it feels good to feel good...doesn't it? It's a good thing...to smile and relax...

Journey on the Path of Abundance

by Dawna Bailey (Hunter)

I'd like you to take a deep breath in...breathing in tranquility, holding for a couple seconds and then exhaling. As you do, allow yourself to feel the calm flowing through your body, and all tensions that you may still hold, being released with your breath as you exhale. And again...taking a wonderful, deep breath in...hold...and release...letting go of all tensions as you drift down...down...into a beautiful state of relaxation and clarity.

Now, I'd like you to visualise, or imagine, just like you do in a daydream, that you are standing at the start of a long corridor...notice how the floor slopes gently downward...easily and gently down toward a door. You can just make out the shape of the door, and that there is a sign on it. You can't quite see what it says yet, though.

Now, start to move...a slow and comfortable stroll...down this long corridor...toward the door. Your steps are easy... graceful...the floor beneath your feet is covered in plush carpet, making every step soft and easy. Down... down...moving closer to the door... feeling totally at ease, as a small thrill of anticipation starts to build at the wonder of what this door holds. Down...and down...closer...and closer.

You are very close now. You can see the sign on the door more clearly. The sign says "Abundance". Take a moment now to imagine what abundance feels like to you. What do you see? What sounds or tastes do you associate with abundance? Is it opulent, or wide? What could lie ahead?

(Pause for 20-30 seconds)

Before you open the door, you notice a sack closed with a long drawstring hanging on the wall next to the door. On the sack you can see the words "Seeds of Abundance" stamped into the fabric. I'd like you to take this sack and comfortably slip it over your shoulder. Now, take another deep breath...feel yourself centre...and as you exhale open the door and step through it.

When you look around you, you notice you are surrounded by a vastness of brilliant, white snow. The air is cold...and crisp. As you breathe in, you can feel the crystal clean air filling your lungs and invigorating you for your journey ahead. You are alive...and vibrant...in this shining sea of snow.

Now, reach into the bag of seeds and scatter a few on the ground next to you...giving thanks for the fresh air filling your lungs, and the reminder of how vibrant and alive you are. Imagine this gratitude nourishing the seeds, as they begin to sprout into an easy path before you...allowing your journey to begin. Walking forward now along this path, taking your time.

And you may notice that you are starting to feel the cold...and just as you notice this, you then notice up ahead next to the path, a large rock. Lying across the rock are warm clothes. As you move forward to the rock, you can see that they are perfectly sized for you. There is a beautiful handmade coat, snow pants, boots and gloves. Each has been created especially for you.

You can allow yourself to put them on. As you dress in these special garments, you notice how soft and warm each is. You notice how light the boots are upon your feet...so easy to move in them. The gloves are soft... yet sturdy. The coat has a full hood that keeps the warmth in, and the cold out. There is even a pair of special glasses to wear...to help reduce the glare of the sun upon the snow...keeping your eyes safe, and comfortable.

Now, reach into the bag of seeds of abundance and scatter a few on the ground next to you...giving thanks for these fine...warm...perfect clothes. These items were made just for you, to keep you safe, and comfortable along your journey. Imagine this gratitude nourishing the seeds...as they begin to sprout and from them animals...gentle in spirit...come forth to populate the vast emptiness that was once there. Their voices begin to quietly, and gently fill the air around you...Their presence is making your journey easier, more tranquil.

You continue forward along the path of abundance, enjoying the comfort of your new clothing, and the ease of the path beneath your feet.

And you may become aware that you are becoming slightly thirsty...and just as you notice this, you see up ahead...a small creek that bends, just to the edge of the path, and then back out...into the snowy wilderness. Sitting on the path is a cup. It is the perfect size to quench your thirst. You can see that the water is clear...clean...sparkling in the sunlight. You may now fill your cup with this water...and drink...deeply. Feel the water ...cool and refreshing...filling you with a sense of perfect clarity, and balance. Feel as the water washes away the thirst, leaving you refreshed...clear...and balanced.

Now, reach into the bag of seeds and scatter a few into the

creek...giving thanks for this gift of fresh water that satiates your thirst, and for infusing you with such beautiful clarity...and balance. Imagine this gratitude nourishing the seeds...as they begin to sprout, and fill the creek with healthy fish to swim playfully through its waters.

You are aware now that these fish are a gift of abundance for you to enjoy. Take a moment to allow yourself to find a quiet pleasure...in their effortless movements through the water...before continuing on your journey.

(*Short pause*)

Good. Now...feeling perfectly refreshed...your mind clear...your whole self balanced... you continue along the path of abundance.

You have been walking a while now, and you may begin to notice that you are growing tired, and you think of how nice it would be to relax. And just as you notice this...you then notice a small cottage up ahead. You can see smoke rising lazily from a stone chimney...being caught and carried away in the breeze. This cottage is the perfect size...no bigger than necessary...just big enough. You walk up to the door and it opens easily as you knock. You walk through the door and find a large table...rustic...inviting. Off to the one side of this little cottage is a beautiful hearth made from the stones of the surrounding land. A warm fire burns steadily and easily within it. You can smell the wood-smoke. You feel the comforting warmth, and listen as the fire pops and crackles. So comfortably at ease, you can now remove all the winter clothing that kept you safe on your journey thus far.

You see a thick, soft chair and ease yourself down into it...reveling in this wonderful relaxation. Beside the chair is a small table for you to place your bag of seeds. And you can just take a nice, deep breath now...inhaling the tranquility and relaxation...exhaling any feelings of exertion. And it feels so good to just relax.

Now, reach into your bag of seeds and scatter a few upon the floor of the cottage...giving thanks for this warm...safe...comforting place to relax. Imagine this gratitude nourishing the seeds...as they begin to sprout, filling the cottage with cherished friends...new...and old. Your heart swells with joy at seeing these friends...growing with a feeling of connection...of sharing...and caring. Love...and harmony...fills the space, and it becomes a home. Take a moment now, to allow yourself to be surrounded with...wrapped in...this glorious sense of love... friendship...harmony...joy.

(*short pause*)

Wonderful.

How beautiful this path of abundance has been so far. For every gift you have been given...you have, in return, taken the time to be aware of it...to return the gift of gratitude...bringing even more abundance to you.

And you may begin to become aware now, that you are becoming a little hungry...and just as you notice this...you notice another door on the far side of the home. You pick up your bag of seeds and walk through it. You are greeted with a garden full of fresh, bountiful foods. The air is warm and ripe with the sweet smells of fresh fruit and earth. Life springs forth in every direction in the vivid colours of nature. Trees laden with fruits and nuts, are plentiful. The branches are easy to reach, and everything in this garden is perfect...healthy...ripe, and ready to be harvested for your meal. Your friends join you in the garden, collecting the foods for a feast. The wonder of abundance surrounds you. The creek full of fish winds its way through this beautiful garden. The birds sing gleefully in the distance. All of the many gifts you have experienced along your path... gather here.

Now, reach into your bag of seeds and take the remaining seeds and spread them all over this beautiful, bountiful garden...giving thanks for the nourishment to your body, your mind, and your inner-self. Imagine this gratitude nourishing the seeds...as they begin to sprout...replenishing all that was harvested for your feast...growing more...and more...growing enough to feed all the creatures, large and small...providing shelter in hard weather...providing homes for the birds and squirrels...providing wood for the fire to keep you warm, and to cook with...giving forth all that is needed, in each and every way.

You return to your friends in the home. They are busy cooking and preparing the feast. The house is alive with abundance from all areas of life. All your needs are met and fulfilled. You want for nothing in this place. You notice over by the fire that there are three pieces of wood. And as you walk over to the hearth, you can see that each piece is carved with a single word.

I would like you now...to pick up one of the pieces. You can see that the word on this piece of wood is Fear. It represents the fear that has blinded you to the abundance that surrounds you at all times, each...and every day. And you can go ahead and throw that piece of wood into the hearth. Watch as it catches fire and burns quickly...the wood charring...turning black...and then into smoke that floats up the chimney, to be caught and carried away on the breeze.

Pick up the second piece of wood, now...You can see clearly that the word on this piece, is Scarcity. It represents all of the times you felt that there wasn't enough to go around...that you must fight, or struggle, to have even the smallest needs met...even though you were...and are...surrounded by abundance at all times. And you can go ahead, and throw that piece of wood into the hearth. Watching as it catches fire and burns quickly...the wood charring...turning black...and then into smoke that floats up the chimney, to be caught and carried away on the breeze

And now I'd like you to pick up the last piece of wood...You can see clearly that the word on this piece, is Lack. It represents the misdirected focus upon what you don't have...it is the distraction that caused you to miss all the gifts that had been offered...it is the sorrow felt when you are lost in want...even though you were...and are...surrounded by abundance at all times. And you can go ahead now, and throw that last piece of wood into the hearth. Watching as it catches fire and burns quickly...the wood charring...turning black...and then into smoke that floats up the chimney, to be caught and carried away on the breeze.

How wonderful it is, to know that you will no longer be burdened by Fear...or Scarcity...or Lack ever again. You can always see abundance now, as it surrounds you every day, and in every way. How amazing your life is now, that you can attract abundance to you...simply by giving gratitude. Doesn't it feel so comforting to know, that your needs will always be met...now that your eyes...and mind, are open to abundance?

And any time you notice those feelings of Fear, Scarcity or Lack trying to creep back in, and blind you to the abundance you seek...you can easily return to this hearth, and throw them in the fire to be burned...releasing you from them, so that you may see clearly and easily the bountiful garden that your path of abundance has led you to.

Now that you are fully aware, and able to give the gift of gratitude through your awareness, you will find it effortless to find new, and creative ways to fulfill all your needs, and wants.

Your friendships will become stronger as you become more open, and grateful for the kindness and connection they offer you. Through your friends, you will find your connections reaching out to more, and more, resources...each new connection helping you to expand even more...opening up even more paths of abundance.

Nothing is outside your reach now.

By being aware...and grateful...for the abundance in your life...you attract more abundance...sowing the seeds of abundance everywhere you go...with everyone you meet.

Negative Baggage Release

by Shona Davenport Blackthorn

Just take a deep breath, hold for count of three and slowly let out any tension and stress.

Now just imagine that you are packing to go on a holiday; you are so excited. Instead of clothes you are packing any baggage, issues, rubbish that you have been carrying around for a long time. Pack everything into suitcases...push them in...sit on them if you can't close the cases...and lock them...

I would like you to imagine calling a cab and telling them you want to be taken to the airport at 3pm or a time that is suitable to your schedule. Now imagine the cab arriving...the cab driver comes to help carry your luggage as you have quite a bit...and it is very heavy. You are on your way to the airport and you are feeling *so* excited...today is *the day* you have been waiting for...for so, so long.

You finally arrive at the airport...the cab driver gets out of the cab, takes your baggage out of the boot of the cab and then finds a trolley for you. Now, you are pushing that heavy trolley into the terminal and you have your boarding pass ready...there are lots of people in front of you and then it is your turn...

The staff member calls to you to come up to their counter...You hand over your boarding pass to the attendant...The attendant asked you to put your baggage onto the weighing scales and you can't help but smile...your baggage being weighed and it is well over the allowed weight and you happily pay the excess weight fee. This is *the day,* and it is worth every extra dollar...

Your baggage begins to disappear on the conveyor belt...moving out of sight...

It's now time to start walking to the number 23 lounge where your flight takes off...

You sit down for a while...relaxing...listening as the boarding call is announced. You then walk over to the window to see your baggage being loaded onto the plane, watch the hatch close and wait for the plane to taxi out and take off...

And then the plane takes off and so does all of that baggage you have been carrying around for so long, out of sight now and gone, gone, gone forever...

What a relief! You can feel yourself straightening up...the weight has gone and now it's time to start a new chapter in your life...

You smile, inside and out, as you begin to imagine how wonderful your life is, without that old, limiting baggage. You feel free, light, relaxed and confident as you stroll out of the airport...now walking into your new, happier life....imagining all of the positive changes that will arrive as a result of this experience...

Congratulations!

The Path

by Heather Lauzon

(*Use your desired induction and deepener*)

I want you to imagine or visualize yourself at a path hidden in a valley. It is a perfect day for a walk. If you have a dog or want a dog you may choose to have it with you now. It is your perfect day so you can make it all that you wish it to be. For you know only you can choose to make each day the best it can be.

You faintly smile at the sight of the inviting path that lies before you, taking a moment to breathe in the crisp coolness of the air that filtered its way through the rainforest. Take in a deep breath...breathing in deep relaxation and exhaling any tension you may feel.

You feel a faint breeze on your cheeks as it pushes its way through the lush fir, cedar and maple trees. Take in a deep cleansing breath, breathing in deep relaxation...and now exhaling any tightness in your body.

The sun is pressing its way through the thick canopy above you, creating playful dancing shadows, as vibrant golden hues pierce through, all around you. It is a perfect day...it is your perfect day.

As you embark down the path, you hear the faint whisper of the breeze as it makes its way through the rich rainforest that surrounds you.

The path winds lazily and easily down, down, down the bank.

The emerald green ferns swaying in the breeze seem to be gracefully waving you on. You notice the tightly curled fronds of young ferns and become aware of how much we are like those tender plants... it is impossible to know or guess what we will be like full-grown when in our early stages of life...and yet we all contain the deep wisdom of Mother Earth.

Our consciousness is awakened through our life experiences. We, like the ferns, are attracted to truth and are drawn to light. We are evolving, surrendering and releasing ourselves along the way to the sure power of light. The fern is Mother Nature's example, an example by creation, that, with patience, one will open itself to the light and flourish steadily into truth.

With this knowledge you now continue down, down, down the trail. A bubbling creek makes itself known to you, where you find a beautiful natural bridge leading you across the creek. You pause at the center of the bridge watching the water flow away from you...arms beside you, palms open. You feel the pull, the gentle tugging of the negative energy from within.

You begin to let go of all anxiety...letting go of all tension...letting go of all fear...allowing the gentle pull to take with it any old beliefs you carry that no longer serve you...Releasing all worries...releasing all self-doubt...very good.

You find yourself simply allowing Mother Nature to take it all and recycle it back into the earth perfectly, and so it is. Take a deep breath in and then breathe deeply out, releasing, releasing, releasing...Very good.

Your hands are down by your side, your palms open. You now turn and face the water flowing as it flows towards you...feeling the gentle flow of positive energy. It almost feels as though it is flowing through you...

Allow this gift from Mother Nature to flow naturally and easily, filling you up with pure positive energy...Inviting and welcoming this gift she has to offer...this gift that fills up with divine pure positive energy. You can feel yourself filling up...filling up with love...filling up with unconditional love...filling up with compassion...filling up with a peace.

As you are standing there, sending out your appreciation and gratitude...you realize you are not alone. Ahead of you...there in the distance stands a Great Blue Heron. You are empowered by its presence...as it shares with you, within your mind, within your soul, that you have the ability to evolve, you can walk with no fear and can stand on your own two feet... and so it is.

As the Great Blue Heron takes you in, you are given the power and energy to be balanced at all times, grounded and centered, and so it is...Reminding you to live in the present, and so it is...Reminding you of your determination and that you are self-sufficient...allowing you to go forward with a quiet mind and a full heart. And so it is....

You turn to leave and you do so...knowing you that you are unique and you have your own unique path...knowing that you will remain strong on your own two feet...with a quiet mind and a full heart.

Finding a Strength Animal

by Camilla Edborg

This can be used for adults and children. It is quite lovely how it helps to bring forward strengths and gives encouraging words. It also helps the client in not feeling alone during the session if need be. (There is a book describing the animals and what they convey called Solöga.)

If there are feelings of darkness, or animal is not friendly, there are some internal disturbances. Take the client away from the scene and proceed with a strengthening script followed by clearing external blocks. (See Page 249)

Gently guide your client to a beautiful meadow, arriving next to a large and beautiful, old apple tree. Let the client sit down comfortably and relax...and breathe in the wonderful air.

(and every breath makes you relax even further, sun is just the way you like it, a gentle breeze making you feel absolutely wonderful and relaxed...etc.)

After a few moments, let the client notice, just a bit further away, that their strength animal is looking forward to coming and meeting them. They will be able to really enjoy this encounter, as it is safe and totally wonderful. Ask what type of animal appears; how it looks, how the eyes feel (*should be loving*), if they want to play with it and hug it, etc. Let them play and have fun.

If they find it loving and strengthening, and if they so desire, it will be with them as we continue along, as company. Suggest if needed, that even if they are awake, they can feel it next to them whenever they would like.

While the client is there, relaxing with their animal, they can play, hug or perhaps share apples from the tree.

This is where I will use other processes, such as an ego strengthening, my *Strength Secret*, or even block removal.

"So... while you enjoy yourself here... you don't need to pay attention to me...I will talk to another part of you...a wonderful part called the subconscious...and I will share a wonderful helpful secret..."

After everything is processed as you have planned, go back to the field with the strength animal(s) and ask the client to express what the animal wants to convey to them...(*write this down*)

Does it have any messages for the client? (*Usually, these are encouraging and with helpful insights...*)

Chapter 11   Helping Children

Confidence Building for School-Age Children

by Sherry Hood

This script is written for elementary school children. It is a general, direct suggestion script that incorporates a small amount of imagery.

You are a very special person. There are many great things about you that make you wonderful. If I began writing them down, it would take a very long time.

Starting today, you can begin being very kind to yourself. I would like you to take time to think about all of the things that make you an interesting person. There are things about you that are so unique and you can begin appreciating all of those things more than ever before.

You like yourself and it shows. Other children can tell that you are comfortable with yourself. They like being around you because it makes them feel good. You smile a lot. You laugh a lot. You have a great sense of humor.

Making people feel happy is one of the special things about you. People love to feel happy and you are very good at this. You can let go of worries. You know that things always work out and you feel confident about that. You decide that worrying only causes you to feel uncomfortable and it really doesn't change a situation, so you are through with worrying.

You can allow yourself to relax and feel so much better because of this.

When you meet new people, whether they are children or adults, you are very confident. You like meeting new and interesting people. When you speak with them, your words flow easily and naturally.

Your posture is great and you are relaxed and calm. You speak clearly. You are comfortable when you are speaking, whether it is to a large group, a small group or to just one other person. You always think of interesting things to talk about. Your mind is clear and it works very well.

No matter what kind of situation you are in, you are relaxed and comfortable. Going to school is a lot of fun for you. You love to learn. Each day is filled with new learning experiences. You do very well in school. You listen carefully to your teachers and you remember everything that is said.

When it is time to do an exam, you are very comfortable and happy, knowing that all of the information that you have been taught is right there in your mind. You do very well on all exams. This helps you to relax and stay calm.

Making friends is easy for you. Other children want to know you. You are interesting and fun to be with. The friends that you make are true friends. You are able to choose the kind of friends that are the best for you.

You sleep very well at night and you always get enough rest and sleep. When you wake up in the morning, you are filled with energy, ready to get up and start your day. Your dream time is always fun and entertaining.

You enjoy staying ahead of things and doing your homework right away becomes a positive habit for you. You are polite and respectful towards your teachers.

You get a lot of exercise, whether it is during gym class, playing at lunch and recess, after school and on weekends. You can see that exercise is very helpful for you. It allows you to be physically fit but it also helps you sleep well at night and exercise helps your body to work properly.

You like to eat healthy foods, including fruits and vegetables. You know that the foods that you put into your body nourish you and help you to grow strong and to stay healthy. You feel so much better when you take good care of yourself.

You are confident, calm and relaxed about everything in your life. People like you and you enjoy being around others. As you go through each school year, you will find that your grades are consistently excellent. This makes you feel very proud because you have worked to make this happen.

Doing well in school is a priority for you. Remember, it doesn't have to be difficult to get good grades. It is natural for you. Before each exam, you picture in your mind the grade that you wish to have. You see it clearly in your mind. You believe that you will get this grade and you tell yourself that it is easy for you to get this grade. Of course, you also need to study and prepare but you feel confident because you have done this. You are learning to use the power of your mind to help you out in all areas of your life.

You are happy, positive, kind and good. You are all of these things and so much more. Every day, you discover new talents and abilities about yourself. You are a fine young person and you will grow into an amazing adult.

Trichotillomania (Hair Pulling) Script for Children

by Ender Tanrikut

This approach contains some aversion technique – use that with discretion.

Imagine that you are in your very own, private movie theater. I wonder if you can see the big movie screen in front of you. On the screen, there is the title of the movie. It says "I stopped pulling my hair." And there is also a picture of you on the screen. It is a happy, smiling picture. It was taken after you stopped pulling your hair. This is why your hair looks healthy and happy; and you look so cheerful and relieved. You did a good job there, I can tell.

Now, please take a moment to notice all the details of the screen; there is no right or wrong. Imagine the screen exactly as you want it to be. Yes, look carefully...

How big is the screen? Where is your picture exactly? On the right side, or the left side, above, or below the title? What color are your clothes? Tell me what else you notice...

You are doing very well...I wonder if you can stay sitting on your chair, and at the same time, imagine yourself doing things I will tell you. This way, you can create your own movie, and watch it in the screen in front of you. If you want you can close your eyes. This way, the movie screen will appear in your mind, and you can watch the movie there.

There is no right or wrong; you can close or open your eyes any time you want. You feel very safe, very comfortable and very, very relaxed.

Let the movie begin:

You are about to go for a walk in the marshmallow park. This is a very safe park, and somebody you love and trust will be sitting beside the park watching you all the time you are there. You can also see that the marshmallow park has two gates; you will enter from one gate, go straight through the wide marshmallow path, and exit from the other gate. The marshmallow park has millions of marshmallows, all soft and fluffy, and in any color you want.

Enter the park. Look around and see and gently touch the marshmallow grass, marshmallow trees, marshmallow leaves, and marshmallow fruits hanging on the trees: apples, cherries, bananas, whatever you like. Take a deep breath and smell the sweet fragrance of the marshmallow flowers. Marshmallows are a little elastic. You can walk or bounce on them. You can bounce very high, and when you hit the ground, the soft and sweet marshmallows help you bounce again. Now I will give you a couple of minutes to walk, bounce and play in the park. (*pause a few minutes*)

Okay. You are getting closer to the exit gate. Now I will start counting from ten to one, and with every number I say, you will bounce once, and with every bounce you will relax more and more. 10,9,8,7,6,5,4,3,2,1.

You've reached the gate, and you are very, very relaxed. Slowly exit the park and imagine yourself sitting on a chair and listening to my voice. When you do this, you feel an urge to pull your hair. You may take time to explore of your feelings. Do you really want to pull your hair? Is that really you who wants to pull your hair, or is it your hand that slowly and forcefully goes towards your hair, like a big, black and hairy spider? Listen. Maybe you can even hear your hand saying with a loud and grumpy voice, "I want to pull your hair, I want to pull your hair...I am coming." Now let it be for a moment, and pay attention to your hair. How is it feeling? Scared, terrified, or intimidated? Can you hear your hair crying and screaming, "Please, please don't hurt me, please (*Name*), protect me!"

You may want to tell your hand to stop hurting your hair. You say, "Stop it!" Oh, it doesn't want stop. Just the opposite: it goes up, and up and up...Your hair looks terrified. Maybe it wants to run away, but it can't because it is fastened to your scalp. You realize that your hands and your hair are parts of your body, and it is your responsibility to take care of them. You know that it is your job to make sure that all your body parts are safe and secure and happy and healthy. You are in charge of your body. You are the boss. You tell your hand again, "Stop it!" But it doesn't listen. It is just being stubborn.

Now, I want you to hold your stubborn hand with your other hand gently, but firmly, so that it cannot pull your hair. At the same time, imagine...just imagine...that your hand is going towards your head, wrapping a string of hair around a finger and pulling it.

Remember, you are not actually doing it. You are holding your stubborn hand with your other hand. At the same time, imagine and feel the stress when your hand pulls your hair. How does your scalp feel? Painful, sore, aching...How do you feel? Maybe relieved, or relaxed...or maybe also embarrassed, or angry...or frustrated...

You may be even feeling guilty...that you weren't able to stop your hand from pulling your hair. But, there is no need for that. I want you to know that it wasn't your fault at all. Your hand was too stubborn and pushy, and you just couldn't stop it. From now on, you will be more firm, and your hand will learn to listen to you.

You did a wonderful job with holding your hand. Until it wants to pull your hair again, you may want to imagine something fun. You could go for a walk in the marshmallow park again. You know that this is a very safe park; the marshmallows love you; and somebody you love and trust is sitting on a bench and watching you. The marshmallow park has two gates; you will enter from one gate, go straight through the wide marshmallow path, and exit from the other gate. The marshmallow park has millions of marshmallows, all soft and fluffy, and in any color you want.

Enter the park. Look around and see and gently touch the marshmallow grass, marshmallow trees, marshmallow leaves, and marshmallow fruits hanging on the trees: apples, cherries, bananas, whatever you like. Take a deep breath and smell the sweet fragrance of the marshmallow flowers. Marshmallows are a little elastic. You can walk or bounce on them. You can bounce very high, and when you hit the ground, the soft and sweet marshmallows help you bounce again. Now I will give you a couple of minutes to walk, bounce and play in the park. (*pause a few minutes*)

Okay. You are getting closer to the exit gate. Now I will start counting from ten to one, and with every number I say, you will bounce once, and with every bounce you will relax more and more. 10,9,8,7,6,5,4,3,2,1.

You've reached the gate, and you are very, very relaxed. Slowly exit the park and imagine yourself sitting on a chair and listening to my voice.

Now you slowly feel the urge to pull your hair again. But this time, you are determined to stop your hand and to protect your hair. It is because you know that your hair deserves your love, appreciation and protection. Your hair loves you; it covers your head to keep it warm in cold winters and cool in hot summers, and it makes you look very handsome (or beautiful). Now it is time for you to show your hair how much you love it by protecting it.

You gently and firmly hold your stubborn hand with your other hand, and imagine saying "Stop it!" or, say quietly, "Stop it." Your hand understands you very well, but tries to disobey you by pushing towards your head. Don't worry, it will listen to you. It is just a little stubborn, that is all. If you want, you may play a trick on your hand by not paying attention to it.

Still holding your hand gently but firmly, just ignore your stubborn hand and imagine doing whatever you would be doing; playing with your favourite toy, eating your lunch or dinner, doing your homework, or watching television. If you need your other hand free, you may occupy your stubborn hand with an important job, such as holding your book, or water bottle, or even keeping it in your pocket until it gives up wanting to pull your hair.

You are doing a wonderful job with managing your hands and your whole body. Your hair feels safe and happy, and very thankful to you for protecting it. Your hand might be a little grumpy at the moment, but actually it is too happy that you lovingly help it become a calm, friendly and gentle hand.

Now I want you to imagine that there is a bright light all around you. It is a very cool and very safe light. It can comfort you, relax you, and heal you. And more importantly, it can also help you and your hand stop pulling your hair. This beautiful, bright light has a golden, white color now, but you can change its color to any other color you wish.

When you breathe, this wonderfully relaxing light will enter your body from your nose or your mouth, go into your lungs, and from there it will travel to every corner of your body to relax it. Every time you take a deep breath, more and more light will enter your body, and stop your hand from wanting to pull your hair.

Now take a deep breath, hold it for a moment and breathe out. Continue breathing deeply; breathe in...breathe out...breathe in...breathe out. This beautiful, loving and relaxing light enters your body, and when all your body is full and glowing with this beautiful light, your hand will calm down, and stop wanting to pull your hair completely.

Breathe in, breathe out...The beautiful light enters your body and flows right to your hands...Your hand calms down a little...feeling safe...feeling loved....

Breathe in, breathe out...More light enters your body and floats all around inside it... from head to hands and to toes...Your hand relaxes more and more....Also, your scalp feels so good, and your hair feels so happy and so safe.

Breathe in, breathe out...More light enters your body...all of your body starts to glow with this beautiful, loving light...It feels pleasantly warm, comforting and very relaxing. Your face, neck, shoulders and arms and hands are relaxing...Your hand is calm, happy, and enjoys itself.

Breathe in, breathe out...More light comes into your body...It flows to your head, to your arms and hands, to your legs and feet, and back to your chest. All of your body is glowing with this beautiful, loving, relaxing and comforting light...Your hand is very happy and relaxed...and gives up bugging your hair.

Breathe in, breathe out...More and more light enters your body...All of your body relaxes more with this beautiful, pleasantly warm feeling...You might feel your body, especially your hands, to be very light, like floating, or heavy; whatever relaxing means to you...

Breathe in, breathe out...More light enters your body, and now your body is full and glowing vividly with this beautiful, loving, comforting, and relaxing light...Your hand is totally relaxed, and feels different; light or maybe heavy, but in each case, very calm and very happy. Your hand stops wanting to pull your hair. It wants to be a gentle and friendly hand.

The beautiful, relaxing and healing light did its job. Now it is time for you to let go. Continue breathing in and out...Every time you breathe out, a little light will go out, but your body will remain relaxed, and your hand will remain calm, and become a friendly and gentle hand.

You did a wonderful job working with the light, and with stopping your hand from pulling your hair. Your hand understands now that you are in charge of your body. It is willing to listen to you, and to become a gentle, friendly hand. From now on, your hand will love and cherish your hair.

There might still be times in that your hand wants to continue its old habit, and pull your hair. If it happens, you need to teach it over and over again to stop doing that, until it finally and completely becomes a gentle and friendly hand.

Now I will give you an anchor. An anchor is a mental tool you can use easily and quickly to relax your hand, and to stop it from pulling your hair.

Every time when your hand wants to pull your hair, I want you to quietly say or think, "Stop it," and hold your hand gently and firmly with your other hand. Don't pay attention to your hand anymore until it relaxes, and gives up wanting to pull your hair.

Every time when you say, or think, "Stop it" to your hand, it will relax faster and easier than the time before, and become more and more a friendly hand.

You did a wonderful job today with creating your own movie where you taught your hand to become gentle and friendly. The movie will stop soon, but your hand will continue being relaxed, gentle and friendly.

In a moment, I will start counting from 1 to 5. When you hear 5, you will fully realize that you are sitting comfortably on a chair in front of me in this beautiful room. You will feel alert, refreshed, relaxed and happy knowing that you stopped pulling your hair.

1...Stop the movie now, and feel the chair beneath you. You can move in the chair, or touch the chair with your hands, and look around if your eyes are open; realize where you are. 2...Look at, or touch your beautiful hand; it feels very relaxed and calm. It finally stopped pulling your hair.

3...Congratulate your hand for stopping to pull your hair. You can hug, stroke or kiss your hand gently. 4...Take a deep breath and have a stretch; you feel so good; you are so happy and relieved that you stopped pulling your hair. 5...You are fully alert, feeling refreshed, energetic and happy.

Congratulations, you stopped pulling your hair!

Chapter 12 Medical and Dental Issues

Auto-Immune Improvement

by Vicky Ortiz

(Originally designed for helping a client who had an immune system problem, along with a needle phobia.)

Everybody is born with an immune system...this is how our body protects itself...When our white blood cells see an intruder in our body...its job is to respond...The white blood cells in the immune system attacks the intruder that invaded our body and destroys it before it can cause any trouble...before it can cause a disease in our body...but sometimes, our immune system makes a mistake...it gets a bit mixed up and attacks a part of our body...by mistake...

Just like one time when I was a kid...about 13 years old, I think...Someone came to my house and I didn't know them...my dog went crazy and wanted to attack the stranger to protect me...My dog was only doing her job...she was being a very good dog, really...but what she didn't know was that the person wasn't really a stranger...and even though *I* didn't know him and my *dog* didn't know him...the stranger actually turned out to be my uncle that was visiting us for the first time...and even though my mom and dad knew him and my dog and I didn't...he really wasn't a stranger after all...my dog just made a mistake...She was really only doing her job...and once we knew that...once my mom introduced my uncle to me and my dog...my dog no longer wanted to attack him...and we all got along just fine...

It's kind of like *your* white blood cells...for some reason they don't recognize your liver...even though your liver is part of your body...just like my uncle was part of my family...your white blood cells can't tell that your liver belongs to you...they've somehow become confused...so, being the good cells that they are, they're trying to protect you from your own liver...That's their job...They're only doing what they're supposed to do...

So now we have to tell them somehow that they need to stop...that you need that liver...that it's your liver and that they need to recognize that it belongs to you...It has to stay...Those cells need to stop attacking it...So how are we going to do that I wonder?...I know...we can go on a quest...

Imagine yourself sitting on the shore looking out at a bright blue sea...it's very sunny and warm out and you feel really happy today...You're throwing rocks into the water...skipping stones...You're walking on the shoreline...at the beach ...You're all by yourself but you feel perfectly happy and content...very safe...no worries at all....

And as you walk...you notice a cave ahead...not too far, but a little ways from you...You're in no hurry...you run along the edge of the water, splashing and jumping...just having fun...maybe remembering the time that you got to fly...thinking it would be cool to do that again...and before you know it, you are at the entrance to the cave...You can feel how cool it feels inside...It would be good to get away from the sun for a while...so hot out here...so nice and cool and refreshing in there...so you let yourself go in...It's not very dark in there....

The opening to the cave is really big and it lets lots of light inside...You know it's all in your imagination anyway and that any adventure you go on will really turn out exactly the way you want it to...just like when you're dreaming...

So you go inside the cave and start to explore...You look at the walls and they're really fuzzy and lumpy and you wonder where the heck you are...It feels really windy in here, too...calm...and then, windy...calm...and then, windy...weird ...and as you look around, you realize that you've somehow shrunk and become really, really small, and that you've walked into your nose!...That's why it's so windy in here, because every time you breathe, it lets the wind in!

You decide to go deeper into your head now...over here is a great big thing that looks like a drum...oh, that must be your eardrum...and over here you can look out of great big round windows...uh huh! This must be your eyes...You walk around and slide down your tongue toward your teeth...oh boy, you really should have brushed better today...

Hey, over there on your lip is some chocolate cake...too big (*person's name*) it's just a crumb, but to mini (*persons' name*), it's the size of a car...yum...You stop to eat a big piece of that chocolate cake...as much as you want...and then you move on...

You walk around in your head until you get to a room with a closed door...that has a sign that says 'brain control room'...DO NOT ENTER...but you know you can enter...it's your brain after all...so you turn the knob and go in...the door's not locked for you...and inside, you find your brain...and it looks like a giant computer...with lights flashing and it looks like it's downloading all kinds of information...wow, talk about super high speed internet!

And there's a scanning machine in there, too...super cool! You step into the glass tube and circles of blue light go up and down your body...it's bright inside the blue light, and it feels warm...you want to see if the scan found anything, so you go to the computer...and you sit down in front of the monitor and you start surfing around...looking at different parts of your body...And then an alarm goes off...really loud...a loudspeaker says, "Warning! Warning! White blood cells are attacking the liver again! Warning!"

Oh, brother, somebody has got to straighten those guys out, and since you're here anyway...you figure you'd better go do it...it is your body after all...

As you explore, you notice red blood cells working hard, carrying their load of oxygen, going all over the place. Those cells start waving and ask, "Hi, (*person's name*), where are you going?" And you reply, "To go straighten out the WBC"...Those red blood cells are pleased, "Great, finally...they sure are causing some trouble!"

On the way you can't resist a stop to jump around, and up and down upon your healthy lungs, soft and spongy...doing belly flops...and then you visit your stomach; oh boy, full of chocolate cake!

And here are your kidneys, hard at work filtering out the junk from your body...

You take a detour over to your left arm and see the switch that *turns off the feeling* to that arm...you think, "That will come in handy for when I get my blood taken...I've got to remember that!"

Finally you arrive at your liver, and it's surrounded by white blood cells...which are acting like big bullies to the liver...

You have a zero tolerance for bullies...no more...it's not nice...You stop to talk to them...they listen because they know you're the boss...and you introduce them to the liver so that they will recognize it from now on...let's all get along now...

The white blood cells say, "Okay, we're sorry. We didn't mean it; we just didn't know. We'll do better..."

On your way back out of your body, you stop at the switch that turns off the feeling to your left arm...and you check out how it works...Every time you flip the switch to OFF, all the feeling to your left arm completely goes away...just like magic...All you have to do is breathe 3 times to relax and then think in your mind about turning off the switch...and just like that, all the feeling in your left arm goes away....

Let's practice it now....don't forget to turn it back on again!

You go back to your head and this time you crawl out of your ear...back out into the sunshine...into the fresh air...And you promise yourself that you will always remember that you have total control of your body...whenever you take 3 deep breaths and think of turning off the switch to your left arm, the feeling in that arm completely goes away...that will come in handy for the days that you have to get your blood taken...

And whenever you think about having to get your blood taken, you think about all the positive results of doing that ...like finding out how well your medication is working for you...Now that you've had a talk with your white blood cells, maybe you won't even still need to take your medication...because maybe one day your blood test will even show that you are all better...that your white blood cells are taking care of your body now...just like you told them to...that your body and your immune system are doing their job, just the way they are supposed to...Now you actually get excited to go get your blood taken...in case today is the day you get the good news...

So instead of getting nervous like you used to...instead of getting sweaty hands...or your head pounding, or the butterflies in your tummy...I don't even know why...you told me that you could never really feel it anyway...instead of getting nervous, now you just take 3 big deep breaths, think of turning off the switch to the left arm...and stay completely relaxed...it's over before you even know it...

Now whenever you have to have a medical procedure and others look at you...they notice how calm you are...In fact, you find that you kind of like the time when you're lying in the bed waiting...because now you can close your eyes and go anywhere you want to...

You can look at the ocean and throw rocks in the water...or walk around inside your body making sure everybody is doing what they're supposed to be doing in there...and you know all about the switch that turns off your left arm...you know about the power of turning off the feeling to that arm...no problem at all....

Return to full awareness, making sure that full sensation is regained in the arm...

Healing Liquid for Pain

by Vanessa Lindgren

Preface this pain relieving process by having the client think of a healing color.

Now we are going to move into our most important and powerful visualization. Do you remember how I mentioned earlier that visualizing things and ideas is very personal?

There are no rules. There is no pressure. You are totally safe and in control. Whatever is in your mind right now is what is supposed to be there. Remember that if I suggest something to visualize, just do your best. If for any reason you can't get a clear picture, try looking at a blank television screen – take your time.

(Therapist takes a long pause)

Actually, *(client's name)* it really doesn't matter at all. You can just go with the flow, you can pretend, you can tune me out, you can feel free to go anywhere in your thoughts because at all times YOU are in control. You can just pretend that you see something, even when you don't. Just pretend...just like a child. It's fine to just pretend.

Now I want you to visualize a beautiful glass. It can be any type of drinking glass that pops into your mind. It can be delicate and ornate; it can be something from your memory. It might be something you own; it could be imaginary...anything, anything at all. Take your time: stay calm and relaxed: take your time to find a glass that looks and feels right for you.

(Therapist takes a long pause)

When you are ready, very comfortably ready, you will raise one finger on your right hand to let me know that you have found a clear visual picture of your glass. There is no rush: stay calm and peaceful: the image will come when you are ready. I can be calm and patient until I see a finger rise on your right hand.

(When finger rises, therapist continues on)

Now I am going to fill your special glass with a clear and crisp liquid. Pure and clean: it's a perfect temperature. Look at your glass now and see the liquid in it. Can you see it? Take your time to see your glass with the pure liquid. When you have a clear image of that, raise a finger on your right hand. You are calm, you are relaxed. Take all the time you need...

(Client's name) That's great. You raised a finger so we are ready to continue our journey.

Now you are going to create the exact color of your liquid. You may have to mix colors to create your special color...

(Therapist now says the color that the client preferred in the pre-talk)

Take your time now. Let your brain do all the work to find the exact mix to make your special color: the color that you can't quite describe in words but you can see in your head...you will know when it's just right. You might think of the little bottles of dye that children use to color their Easter eggs...you know that food safe dye that is safe to eat or drink just like coloring the icing on a birthday cake. Your mind will mix the dyes to create that special color you told me about.

It takes just the precise touch...you'll know when it's exactly right. I can wait patiently until you've mixed the color perfectly...when you are ready, raise a finger on your right hand.

Now take about three big sips of your healing liquid. I will know when you have swallowed a few sips because I will see your throat move just a little.

(Therapist waits to see the swallow in the throat)

Your healing liquid is now travelling calmly and swiftly through your body. Do you remember ever looking at one of those diagrams in a biology book where you see a figure standing with arms stretched out? You know...like a school biology book or something. A simple picture where you can see all the veins, muscles, organs and all the body parts. Find that picture now...I'll wait. You can always look at your TV screen if you need help capturing this image. I'll wait...there's no hurry. Raise one finger on your right hand when you have a clear picture of the inside of a body.

Now see your entire body flooded with your special healing liquid; that gorgeous color you have created.

(Therapist says the color)

It is filling your veins. It is mixing perfectly with all your body fluids and travelling to every part of your body. Organs, muscles, nerves, nerve receptors, ligaments, bones, tissues, cells...everywhere; no matter how miniscule a capillary of part of your body might be, it is now beautifully flooded with your healing liquid. It is melting away the pain...it knows exactly where you feel pain...it knows exactly where the source of the pain is. It can seek and destroy the pain.

It melts it away effortlessly...it is way more powerful than the pain...your special healing liquid has all the knowledge it needs to find anything in your body that needs repair; that needs attention. It is melting the hurt, it is melting the pain away...

I want you to know that when you are in pain you can simply pick up your glass and drink more of your special healing liquid. Anywhere, anytime. Your subconscious knows about your liquid; it knows when you need another dose, it knows where it must travel.

If you forget to take extra liquid when you're in pain, don't worry. You took several sips today and that will be in your body forever. Travelling around and melting the pain; seeking and destroying the pain. You have really turned a corner today with your pain...with controlling your pain.

Feel safe, feel calm. Enjoy the relief. Feel the relief. You have so much relief from your pain...

Tumor Breakdown – Healing Soldiers

by Doris Santic

I find tumors are becoming more and more common these days and I believe it has everything to do with "Nursing old hurts and shocks...building remorse." I think these people need help to "lovingly release the past and turn their attention to this new day."

For the Visual Client:

Visualize or imagine a group of soldiers on their way to help you...YOU are not alone! Look at them...there's SO MANY of them...who care about YOU...and want to help...because they LOVE YOU...Watch as they come closer and closer towards you...See these soldiers...organized in MANY rows...wearing GORGEOUS white uniforms with gold buttons....because they are SPECIAL healing soldiers....You see...as they get closer...some soldiers are holding instruments...BEAUTIFUL shiny instruments made of gold...As they get closer...you see...they are playing YOU a song...

Some other soldiers...are pulling an object behind them...It looks like some sort of machine...being carried on wheels... NOTICE the look on their faces...they are SO excited and happy...to be able to do this for YOU...As they reach you now...they know EXACTLY where the tumor is located...and set up shop right next to it...These fabulous soldiers have done this MANY times before...and are AWESOME at working together...

You watch...as they prepare what they need to do...and it's VERY interesting to see...It looks like the machine is a laser...and they have brought it...to breakdown the

345

tumor...This machine puts out...the MOST BEAUTIFUL color of WHITE in its beam...SO white and SO pure...SO full of color...it's actually GLOWING...You watch...as they point their laser at the tumor...and just KNOW that YOU are perfectly SAFE...These soldiers have come to help YOU...and they do their jobs well...You see the laser is working...because pieces are falling off NOW...SO effortlessly...SO easily...and it feels SO GOOD to see this...NOTICE many of the soldiers begin to pick up...and carry the smaller broken pieces...while YOU watch...the rest of the tumor...being broken up further...NOW...

What color is the tumor?...Does it have a texture?...What does it look like to YOU?...Watch as they blast the LAST bit of tumor...into many tiny little pieces...so that they're small enough for the soldiers to carry...Now...ALL the soldiers gather together briefly...to make a plan for the route OUT...They KNOW that ALL remnants of the tumor have to be taken OUTSIDE of your body....in order for you to HEAL FASTER...Watch them carry the tiny pieces strategically ...You see a trail of white light...as you watch the soldiers...get further and further AWAY...This light has been left behind for YOU...because it will...CONTINUE to help you HEAL quickly...This light helps HEAL EVERYTHING that is necessary to balance you PERFECTLY in EVERY way...These soldiers LOVE their work...and they LOVE YOU...and they want YOU to ENJOY life...

You NOW realize...the past doesn't matter anymore...and you look forward to the future...BUT you have LEARNED to FOCUS on living in the PRESENT moment...now and always...Each day...Each hour...and Every minute...letting the past go...not worrying about the future...just BEING and living in the PRESENT moment...The need for remorse is gone...you have paid your dues...You RELEASE the need to feel stuck in deep and painful regret...

You are NOW FREE...What do you see in your life as you

heal, and then after...What do you visualize around you...What does your perfect life look like?

For the Auditory Client:

Imagine a group of soldiers on their way to help you...YOU are not alone! You hear footsteps coming towards YOU...it sounds like...there are SO MANY of them...who care about YOU...and want to help...because they LOVE YOU...Listen carefully...as they come closer...and closer towards you...The soldiers are marching...in MANY rows...in PERFECT rhythm...to the BEAT of the drums...Some soldiers are holding instruments...amazing instruments made of gold...They play a BEAUTIFUL song for YOU...You listen JOYFULLY...as they play their song for YOU...These soldiers sing in PERFECT harmony...You say to yourself...these are SPECIAL healing soldiers...and you realize...they have come to help YOU HEAL...The HAPPY cheers...of the EXCITED soldiers...get louder as they come closer...They are SO happy to be able to do this for YOU...

As they get even closer...you hear something being pulled behind them...they call it some sort of healing machine...it's being carried on wheels...As they reach you NOW...they know EXACTLY where the tumor is located...and you hear them setting up shop right next to it...These fabulous soldiers have done this MANY times before...and are AWESOME at working together...You hear some noise...as they prepare what they need to do...and it's VERY interesting to listen to...

It seems that this machine is a laser...and they have brought it...to help breakdown the tumor...This machine puts out...the MOST BEAUTIFUL sound while the beam is turned on...SO pure...SO heavenly...like angels singing...a tune like you've NEVER heard BEFORE...You listen carefully...as one of the soldiers tells you...that you are perfectly SAFE....You call out to a soldier...standing next to the laser...and tell him that you ARE READY to begin...

347

You rest and listen....while the soldiers begin to work...hearing that tune...that fabulous tune...that you could listen to for an eternity...As they point that laser to the tumor...you hear the laser beam hitting the tumor...notice the sound...as the pieces begin breaking apart...you hear the laser working...These soldiers have come to help YOU...and they do their jobs WELL...SO effortlessly...SO easily...and it feels SO GOOD to hear all this...NOTICE many of the soldiers begin to pick up...and carry the smaller broken pieces...while YOU listen...the rest of the tumor...being broken up further NOW...Do you want to say something to the tumor before it's GONE...What do you need to discuss to feel harmonious... Now is the time to speak up and be heard...Listen as they blast the LAST bit of tumor...into many TINY little pieces...so that they're small enough for the soldiers to carry...Now...ALL the soldiers gather together briefly...to discuss a plan for the route OUT...They KNOW that ALL remnants of the tumor have to be taken OUTSIDE of your body...in order for you to HEAL FASTER...Listen as they carry the tiny pieces strategically...As you say GOODBYE to the soldiers beginning to leave...

You thank them for all of their help...and tell them how grateful you are for their love...you listen...as the familiar footsteps...get further and further AWAY...You hear that angelic tune again as the soldiers carry the pieces OUT of your body...Their song is within you now...and it helps HEAL EVERYTHING that is necessary to balance you PERFECTLY in EVERY way...These soldiers LOVE their work...and they LOVE YOU...and they want YOU to ENJOY life...

You NOW realize...the past doesn't matter anymore...and you look forward to the future...But you have LEARNED to FOCUS on living in the present moment...now and always...Each day...Each hour...and Every minute... letting the past go....not worrying about the future...just BEING and living in the PRESENT moment...The need for remorse is gone...you have paid your dues...You RELEASE the need to feel stuck in deep and painful regret...You are NOW FREE...What do you hear happening as you heal...and then after? How does the end result sound to you? What do you want to hear people saying?

For the Kinesthetic Client:

Imagine a group of soldiers on their way to help you...you are not alone...You feel there are SO MANY of them...who care about YOU...and want to help...because they LOVE YOU...You can feel their presence getting stronger...as they get closer and closer towards you...It's all SO real...ALL these soldiers...organized in MANY rows...You feel the LOVE...from all these soldiers...who are coming in to help YOU...you are SO happy and grateful...that you are not alone...You feel the most POSITIVE emotions just being around them...because they are SPECIAL healing soldiers...You notice as they come closer...that some are holding instruments...BEAUTIFUL instruments made of gold...As they get closer...you feel humbled by the song they play just for YOU...You can feel ALL the love in their song...Some of the soldiers are pulling something behind them...you are VERY curious to what it is...

It seems like some sort of machine...being carried on wheels...NOTICE the look on their faces...they feel SO excited and happy to be able to do this for YOU...As they reach you now...you can feel your own excitement building...as you wonder what will happen next...The pressure is almost too much...but you TRUST them because you know they LOVE YOU...so you are able to go with the flow...They know EXACTLY where the tumor is located...and set up shop right next to it...These fabulous soldiers have done this MANY times before...and are AWESOME at working together...You feel VERY relaxed as they prepare the things they need to do...and it's very calming to know they are here...

It turns OUT the machine is a laser...and they have brought

349

it...to help breakdown the tumor...This machine...puts out the most BEAUTIFUL vibration...when the beam is turned on...SO pure....SO warm...SO VERY comfortable...Although you have just met...you TRUST them thoroughly...and feel extremely SAFE...They can sense that you're ready...so they begin to point the laser at the tumor...as you feel this WONDERFUL sense of relaxation...a sensation like you've never felt...this feeling warms up your entire body...and it feels SO GOOD...You feel more COMFORTABLE than you have ever felt...SO loved...SO warm...SO VERY comfortable..These soldiers have come to help YOU...and they do their jobs WELL...You can sense the laser is working...because you feel lighter...as the laser beam breaks down the tumor into smaller pieces...you may smell smoke as pieces are broken up further...SO effortlessly...SO easily...and it feels SO GOOD to feel this way...you notice many soldiers pick up the small pieces... and begin to carry them away...causing you to feel lighter and lighter...as these pieces begin to be moved OUT and AWAY from your body...Leaving you feeling PERFECTLY calm and relaxed...happy and excited...grateful and humbled...

What does the tumor feel like to you?...How does it touch your life?...Feel them blast the LAST of the tumor NOW...into many TINY little pieces...so that they're small enough for the soldiers to carry...Now ALL the soldiers gather together briefly...to find the best route OUT...They KNOW that ALL remnants of the tumor...have to be taken OUTSIDE of your body...in order for them to feel you will HEAL FASTER...You are in awe...as you watch them move out ALL the small pieces strategically...As you sense the soldiers...getting further and further AWAY...you notice the 'feeling of healing' is left within you...long after they are GONE...because it WILL continue to help you HEAL quickly...This 'feeling of healing' helps HEAL EVERYTHING that is necessary to balance you PERFECTLY in EVERY way...These soldiers LOVE their work...and they LOVE YOU...and they want you to ENJOY life...

You NOW realize...the past doesn't matter anymore...and you look forward to the future...BUT you have LEARNED to FOCUS on living in the PRESENT moment...Each day...Each hour...and EVERY minute...letting the past go....not worrying about the future...just BEING and living in the PRESENT moment...The need for remorse is gone...you have paid your dues...You RELEASE the need to feel stuck in deep and painful regret...You are NOW FREE!!!

What do you feel happening as you heal...and then after? Do you feel the most POSITIVE emotions when you reach the end result? How does this touch your life? What does your perfect life feel like to you?

Relaxing through Your MRI

By Seth-Deborah Roth

Now just allow yourself to relax. Go ahead and close your eyes. Allow yourself to relax and let all the little muscles of your eyes relax...Now take a deep breath and exhale. Allow yourself to settle in and feel real comfortable as you concentrate on breathing in and breathing out. Belly button going out as you inhale and going belly button going in as you exhaled...Breathing in and breathing out...Relax and release...Relax and release...Feeling the muscles around your eyes start to relax even more. Imagine...allowing your eyes start to feel heavier and heavier – so heavy that they feel as if they are glued shut or some liquid wax has just melted them closed. You know you could open them if you wanted to but you just don't want to. They feel so good being closed,, so heavy...so relaxed. If your eyes start fluttering or feel as if they are moving around, that's okay. Just keep them shut and listen to the words. You may want to let my words help make pictures in your imagination or just give you a sense of relaxation.

Taking some deep breaths now, real slow. Feel your breathing slowing down. Feel your breathing slowing down. And as you keep your eyes closed and let your body relax, you may feel a gentle, peaceful wave of relaxing energy, like a waterfall going from the top of your head all the way down to your toes. A gentle wave of relaxing energy is helping you to relax all the way from your head down to your toes. Allow yourself to pretend that you have just become a Raggedy Ann or Raggedy Andy doll. You know the old kind of rag dolls that just flop around. They look as if they don't have any bones. They just flop around and look raggedy...Now I want you to pretend that you have just become one of those rag dolls. So your arms have become loose and limp. Just loose and limp like an old rag doll. Your arms are all limp and your legs are all limp. You are just lying here feeling very loose and limp. Your breathing is very relaxed...Real slow...Breathing in and breathing out. Real slow...Very good. Feeling really good...

In the background, you may hear the tapping of the MRI machine. You hear the rhythm of the tapping. The rhythm of the tapping just makes you get more and more relaxed as you hear it in the background. Every time you hear the rhythm of the tapping, you allow yourself to get more and more relaxed. You get so relaxed with the tapping in the background that it actually seems to fade away like white noise just fading away in the background. The sound of the tapping just reinforces the knowing that you are taking care of your body and will get the answers that you need. This knowledge just makes you feel better and better about this test. The knowledge that you will soon receive your answers and your information just makes you feel better and better about this test.

Now allow your body to begin to feel kind of heavy. And feel your body sinking into the gravity of the earth. Feel your body sinking into the gravity of the earth. Just allow it to happen and feel your body sinking into the gravity of the earth. You arms are real limp and heavy. And your legs are kind of heavy and limp now. You don't feel like moving any part of your body. Your body feels heavier and heavier, so easy staying in one position. Heavier and heavier, so easy staying in one position...And you are real comfortable and real relaxed, controlling the relaxation in your muscles, feeling at ease and physically relaxed...So easy and so in control...staying in one position.

Controlling the relaxation in your muscles, feeling at ease and physically relaxed...So easy and so in control...staying in one position.

And now that you are physically relaxed, I'd like you to just allow your mind to relax, remembering that you are in total control. You have allowed yourself to relax physically and now you allow yourself to mentally relax. You are in total control. You have allowed yourself to physically relax. And now you can mentally relax.

In a moment, not yet, but in just a moment, I'm going to count down from 25 to 1. With each number, you will be able to mentally relax and allow yourself to go deeper and deeper into relaxation. Some people see the numbers. Some people feel the numbers or just imagine the numbers. Whichever you do is just fine. You may find that you will be able to double your relaxation with each number as you go deeper and deeper into relaxation.

25, 24, 23. Feeling more and more relaxed.

22, 21, and 20. Doubling your relaxation.

19, 18, 17. More and more relaxed. Feel the relaxation.

16 and 15. Once again, allowing yourself to double the relaxation. Very good.

14. Deeper and deeper with each exhalation.

13, 12, 11, and 10. Once again, doubling your relaxation.

9. Just letting the relaxation and the stillness happen.

8, 7. That's it. Letting yourself go deeper. More and more relaxed.

6, 5. Once again, doubling your relaxation. Letting it happen.

4. Staying still and perhaps doubling your relaxation again knowing that you are in control and letting it happen.

3, 2, and 1. Deeply relaxed. Being very, very still. Just relaxing. Being very, very still and just relaxing.

When the test is completed and the technician brings you out of the MRI machine, you count up from 1 to 5. And on the number 5, you open up your eyes feeling alert, and energized, and knowing that you have taken an important step to optimal health.

Relief from Bruxism (Night Grinding)

by Bev Bryant

Right now...I'd like to suggest that you get into a comfortable position and relax...it doesn't matter if you are sitting in a chair, or laying down on a couch, bed or floor...just relax and allow your mind to listen to the sound of my voice as you are becoming even more aware of the music...you already know there is nothing you need to do right now as you drift along listening to the music and becoming even more aware of your breathing...knowing that if at any time while you are listening to this, if there is anything you need to attend to...you will be able to open your eyes, become wide aware and tend to your business...now... take a deep breath...hold it...let it release...now take another deep breath...hold it...hold it and let that one go too...releasing any and all tensions as you are breathing out... paying attention to your breathing...with every breath you take... and every word I speak, allowing yourself   just   to   relax   even more...good...begin counting down from 10 to 1...slowly ...seeing the numbers in your mind ... you imagine them as I continue talking... you just keep counting...relaxing more and more with every breath you take....and you can choose to listen to my voice or your mind may wander...whatever you do being just the right thing for you to do at this time...that's right...relaxing deeper and deeper with every breath you take...knowing you are doing something special just for you....

Noticing just how relaxed you become already, and we've just begun...that special relaxed way about you that only you know about...the way you can relax your feet...maybe even feeling a tingling sensation in your toes...as this feeling moves up your legs now feeling so good...so calm...so relaxed as it moves to your thighs...total relaxation for your legs now...and I'm wondering if that tingling sensation has moved there also...as your torso relaxes now...your stomach...your chest and your back...relaxing your spine...just letting go and just maybe you feel that tingling sensation move up and down your spine...relaxing your shoulders...just feeling your shoulders relaxing on down...as your neck now becomes so relaxed that you just can't help but feel your head going deeper and deeper into whatever it is relaxing upon... feeling the muscles in your face and scalp relaxing on down in their own special way...right down to the tiniest muscles in the forehead...the eyes...the nose... cheeks...and ears....

And as we get to the mouth and jaw...you may feel that special tingling sensation as you discover a special way to relax that part of you that seems almost magical...only you know about this total relaxation for your mouth and jaw...even your teeth and tongue feel relaxed....you can even feel the back of your tongue relaxing...it may even be hard to hold your lips together now...and it's ok if your lips part in their own special relaxed position...going deeper and deeper...now that's total relaxation...and each time you listen to this you will find yourself going much deeper and more relaxed...calm...feeling so good...and you know when you feel this way your body normalizes clear down to the cellular level...tapping into your inner calm and strength...your mind and body can do magical things in this state of relaxation in a short amount of time...emotionally...mentally...and physically ...

Now...I'm wondering if you can imagine a magical place that you can go to.... a very special place where you can go to in your mind where you feel safe, secure, and relaxed...now...this place can be inside or it can be outside...it doesn't matter...a place where your mind can take you anytime you feel the need to relax...now notice everything around this place...maybe if you imagine it is in color...the colors are very vibrant...there could be a warm soft breeze...notice any sounds ...or smells...and as you are looking around, feeling wonderfully relaxed and safe...you may even see an inviting place to sit or lay down...so you go there now and sit or lay down...maybe you close your eyes and can feel the sun on your face...and you somehow know that this is where you can go to get answers...all you have to do is ask and the answers come to you...

It's beautiful here...and there's a part of you that knew the answers were there all along...you just had to ask...you might ask why you grind your teeth at night...or clench them during the day....having that answer could relax those muscles forever...or, you could ask that a special mentor or spiritual being to be there with you and that can help you to come up with the answers...someone you know that has all the answers...now...you can come to this special magical place anytime you like...you can be there alone or you may invite whoever you like...now... here's the secret in going to your special place...you simply close your eyes... take a deep breath...and as you exhale you say to yourself, relax... and you are there...now...I want you to imagine yourself in a typical stressful situation...at work, at home, with the kids, whatever it may be...and find a place you can go be by yourself for a minute...perhaps it's a bathroom...a bedroom...your car...wherever you can be by yourself...be there...and closing your eyes...taking a deep breath...and as you are exhaling you say to yourself relax...and you are in your special magical place...and you may find you may only need to be there for a few minutes and you are completely relaxed and ready to take life on again...that's right...

I would like for you to practice this one more time...so I will be silent while you practice ...that's right...(*long pause*)...good...that's right...now that you know how to practice that one...and while you are relaxing in your special place, going deeper and deeper...there is one more thing I would like you to practice...now this would be a good thing for you to do when you go to bed at night...so picture and imagine yourself walking to your bed and notice how good it is going to feel when your head reaches the pillow...this is all you care about right now as you are getting ready to climb in your bed...as you get into your bed you may already know then your head hits your pillow it is your signal to relax... especially your jaw muscles and all those tiny muscles around your mouth...it feels so good...and its ok if your lips part in their own natural way...remembering how relaxed you are right now...you already know that's how it is going to be every time your head hits the pillow...and you may even go to your special place where there is total relaxation...and while you are sleeping...if your muscles around your jaw area start to tighten...that will be the signal to your subconscious mind to relax all those muscles even more...that's right...relaxing them even more...now...

I want you to practice picturing and imagining yourself going to bed...feeling your head gently begin to relax on the pillow and notice how your jaw muscles instantly relax...you may not even know this is happening consciously...that doesn't matter... as long as your subconscious knows...your subconscious mind is what takes over when we are sleeping anyway....so go ahead and practice that now...(pause)...that's right...let your subconscious tell all the muscles around your mouth to just let go...it's ok to just let go...and let this new useful pattern replace the old unwanted pattern that was there before...letting your sleep become restful and refreshing every night...that is where your body loves to go...to that special place where there is magical total relaxation...enjoying the sensations now as you feel this encompass your whole body...

You may even remember a time when you were young and your sleep was so natural...no worries....letting your subconscious acquaint you with your new pattern in its own gentle, soothing way...just the right way for you...and your subconscious knows exactly what that is...letting yourself become curious...so it becomes easy now for this to happen...as you go deeper and deeper relaxed...enjoying the feeling more and more...knowing you are doing something good just for you...as this feeling relaxes you even more...that's right...relaxing you even more...you never knew you could become so relaxed...but it was there all along...inside you all along...or were you inside it...now it can stay there so you may enjoy it every night...wouldn't it wonderful to be able to enjoy this every night?...

Now...you have learned that your mind and body work together...synthesizing everything to a perfect rhythm...tune into it now...and, knowing your subconscious can make your heart beat at regular intervals without the conscious mind being involved...every body part flowing at its own natural pace.... the central nervous system flowing smoothly now that your body and mind have shared this information...looking forward to putting into use what you now know...and if this was there all along...looking forward in discovering what else there is to discover...

I would like you to notice something in your future...something that would show you just how well this has worked for you...maybe it's how much better you are sleeping at night ...maybe it's noticing how relaxed you are upon awakening...maybe it's noticing how it is much easier to cope with stressful situations, remembering to use self-hypnosis whenever you need it...that's right...noticing how good your teeth feel...your gums are pink and healthy...your jaw in total relaxation...noticing the old unwanted symptoms you used to have are no longer there...that's right...replaced by the new pattern your subconscious has developed...you may even remember successes you have had in the past and because you have had those successes in the past it's easy to imagine how they make you feel...it's ok to remind yourself of the successes you have had in the past...and how those successes give you confidence for this success in the future...and future successes in the future...and noticing how good that makes you feel...it's okay to allow yourself to feel proud...maybe other people are noticing how much more relaxed you are and are giving you compliments...as your subconscious shows you just how well this has worked for you...

Notice how powerful you truly are...and how all this power is coming from within you...recognize this within yourself...acknowledge yourself...yes, this is coming from within you...feel how good it feels...and how positive change can come so easily for you now...thinking of all you have learned and experienced now...go ahead and reinforce it...let your subconscious tell your conscious mind that this is ok...and how much better you feel...now you know exactly what to do...where to put your focus when you need to...and you know it extremely well...

Now...if this is your normal sleep time...go ahead and fall gently and deeply asleep...deeper than you ever have before...accepting all things that are for your highest good...making them a new and improved way of life for you...and it feels so good to be doing that special something just for you...remembering to just let go...that's right...just letting go...and if you need to become wide aware and rested...I am going to count you up now...so when you hear the number 10...you will become wide aware and feel rested, relaxed and ready to take on the rest of the day...

1...remembering to do your self-hypnosis whenever needed...simply taking a deep breath and saying relax and allowing yourself to go there...2...just going to that safe place at the appropriate time and place...3...remembering how special you are...you may even become pleasantly surprised at your ongoing progress...4...paying attention to your body and jaw... relaxing and releasing it at the appropriate times...5...noticing how good a smile feels...6...when your head hits the pillow tonight it feels so good...7... your ability to relax becoming easier and easier ...8... beginning to notice whatever you are sitting or lying upon ...9...when you open your eyes they feel refreshed...10...opening your eyes...taking a deep breath...returning to full awareness...feeling great...

Arterial Metaphors for Circulatory Improvement

by Kelley T. Woods

I created this to help a diabetic build new peripheral arteries but is suitable for anyone suffering from circulatory impairment. Use this once your client has been taught and has mastered stress management and pain control technique. I use a conversational hypnosis approach which quickly moves into a fully engaged trance as the client's imagination is harnessed!

1. Calibrate pain awareness level; adjust to tolerable level (Even better, gage comfort level!)

2. Discuss circulatory system as a transportation system within the body: powered by the engine (heart), the blood cells and fluids use the arteries (freeways) to travel out of the heart to the various points...ending at the capillaries (turnarounds)...

Have the client open and close a fist one time each second to demonstrate this is the rate of that engine pumping. Explain that it takes about 60 of these pumps to circulate the total amount of blood throughout the body when at rest like the client is right now.

Along the way, the job of the arterials is to allow the blood to move smoothly and easily and to be able to drop off its deliveries of oxygen and nutrients. This smooth delivery requires that the arterials be clog-free and flexible, without ruts or barriers of any kind. Explain that the conditions of the roads can be affected by many different influences, such as stress, diet, genes...that any built up materials alongside the roads or even in the roadway are like unwanted litter that can hinder the movement of the traffic.

Include sub-modality of color by explaining that oxygen-rich blood from the heart is bright red and as it travels to the extremities and then back through the veins to the engine, it changes color to blue. On the way back to the engine, the blood removes waste product, making the return journey just as vital. Of course, the client knows how important it is to re-oxygenize the blood by breathing deeply, by keeping the lungs healthy and clear, by managing stress and tension to allow better breathing, etc.

3. Calibrate the "traffic flow" of the client's blood. Mention the sub-modalities involved in the rate: artery quality (width, flexibility, congestion), oxygen level (color) and give time for the client to consider these. Ask what speed that blood is now moving through the highways from the heart, with 1 being the lowest, most sluggish rate and 10 being the most healthy, healing goal rate.

4. Begin the imagery of the client's circulatory system as a freeway network. Have the client visualize a collection of blood cells, both red and white, as they are "fueled" with oxygen and then pumped back into the network. Drop the client into the collection, as if the collection is a vehicle of sorts. Let the client describe the type of vehicle he is "driving", using somatic references for his experience.

5. Allow the client to witness the condition of the "freeway", including any details that he notices such as the quality of the road surface, any restrictions or barriers, widening or narrowing of the shoulders, etc. Lead the client to some areas

that are more restrictive and uncomfortable than others and track the rate of speed as it varies. Notice any changes in the client as he experiences these; how he reacts to the different sub-modalities.

6. From the most restrictive place, release the client to imagery of wide, open country lanes, likening them perhaps to an appropriate geographical reference...where there are no speed limits, no traffic, no dead ends or constrictions or restrictions, etc...Allow plenty of time for the client to enjoy and process this sense of circulatory freedom, circling around every minute or so, letting him notice that each cycle becomes easier and easier. The road is opening wider and more comfortably with each pass.

7. The return trip to the heart is through the veins. This is the time to address key emotional components that may be influencing your client here by allowing them to "lighten" the load of their vehicles by depositing these unwanted emotions into the traffic blood flow, letting them be carried away with the rest of the waste.

8. Allow the client as many trips through his network as he needs to make the change work in his blood traffic flow. Calibrate with every pass.

9. Conclude the imagery with allowing the client to float out of his circulatory vehicle and reintegrate with his body in your presence. Run an ecology check and ascertain with parts that the client experienced a change and is able to re-connect with that process on his own.

10. Include suggestions for attendance to practicing not only this imagery daily, but staying on course for healing through regular stress management technique.

Chronic Pain

By Birgit Wujcik

I want you to know that I have helped many people reduce their pain and I feel confident that together we can change and reduce the pain you have suffered for so long.

Have you ever put any thought into all the different sensations that your body experiences? When you really think about it there are many pleasant and unpleasant sensations that we experience on a daily basis.

Sensations are a way for our body to communicate with our mind. A good sensation might bring about pleasure and trigger happiness, peace and joy. A bad sensation might feel unpleasant and generate feelings of anger, helplessness and despair. The outcomes of both good and bad sensations are stored in your mind to be recalled when necessary at a later date.

All sensations have a purpose. They are a way for you to know what is really going on so that you can take action.

Imagine not having any sensation at all...You would not know when you are hurt or when you are approaching your limit of an activity. You would not know if something was good for your body or bad. How would your mind store any important information for you to learn and grow?

I would like to invite you to close your eyes for just a moment. Perhaps you may want to leave your eyes closed for the time being but it does not matter.

As you are comfortably breathing in and out I would like you to pay attention to your sensations right now...

How do your hands feel as they are resting comfortably beside you? What sensations do you experience in your hands right now? Do they feel light or heavy? Warm or cold? Are your palms dry or moist? Are your fingers touching and how does the material of the chair feel on your skin?

As you are focusing on the sensation of you hands you may not have paid any attention to your feet but by mentioning your feet now...your mind immediately scans all information pertaining to the sensation in your feet. It just happens...this process works so fast that in a split second you are provided with all the information necessary to make a decision. So, as you are now focusing on the sensation of your feet I would like to invite you to let go of any tension that you may be holding onto...allowing your muscles to go loose and limp. Allowing all muscles in your body to release, smooth out and relax...ahhh...That feels so good ...doesn't it?...As you do that, your body is sending information about all areas to your mind right now.

There are some areas that are very easy to relax as the sensation is pleasant and there is no threat or danger to be hurt...

The reason that you are here is because you are experiencing pain in a very special area (*insert client's personal information about pain*).

Your body is communicating that there is something wrong. That is the purpose of pain...to let you know when you need to take action – if you don't take action or if you do not change the situation your body responds with more pain...until the problem is fixed. Does that make sense?

So really, we should be thankful for pain signals to alert us that there is something wrong...You may thank your body right now in the privacy of your mind for doing such a great job. You are perfect in every way...Every sensation that you experience is for your benefit...

As you focus on the pain right now, thanking your body for letting you know that there is a problem, notice that the intensity of the pain is stronger as you focus on it. This makes perfect sense...Just imagine your body sending out signals all the time...over and over...and nothing happens...and then...finally you pay attention...it's like a jump for joy as your (*insert client's area of pain*) finally gets looked at and cared for.

But you know that this signal has no longer a purpose if the damage is permanent and chronic. The pain signal is only meaningful if you can change the condition to allow your body to heal. You have done the very best you can...(*insert all treatment, surgery, medications, physiotherapy , activity, lifestyle change etc. that client has undergone or performed*) and now it is time to change the perception of the pain that you are experiencing. Yes, your body will continue to send messages to your mind but you know that those messages no longer have a meaningful purpose...So you can change how you feel about those sensations...

There are many ways to change how you perceive pain and this is just one of many ways to allow you to continue living a full and enjoyable life or perhaps to regain your independence and freedom. Sometimes you need to test out different approaches in order to find the one that works best for you...like trying on new shoes...they are all the same size of shoes and yet not all of them feel right...You have taken many different medications for your pain and have attempted many different strategies to cope...so let's begin and see how well this approach fits you...

On a scale of 0 – 10...0 being no pain at all and 10 being the worst pain you have ever experienced, where would you say your pain is right now? (*write down client's response*)

As you focus on your pain right now. I would like you to take in a deep breath and gently allow all of the muscles around the area of your pain to relax. That's right...take in another breath and as you breathe out, relax those muscles around the area a little more...

Now I want you to describe what you are experiencing...the pain, as it is...describe it the best way you can. (*allow client to formulate a description*)

If you had magic powers, how would you change this pain around so that you can tolerate it ? At what level would your pain need to be so that you can live your life to the fullest, able to enjoy many things?

(*If client stumbles or is searching...suggest:*)

Perhaps I can help you with this...When you look at the pain with your inner eye, how does it look like? Does it have a color or a shape? What is it made of?

If you could make it an object, what would it be? How big is it and where exactly is it...more to the front or right in the middle or perhaps in the back? Is it under the skin or right on top?

Perhaps there is a sound to the pain...or maybe a smell? Is the pain solid or liquid or squishy? Does it have a taste to it?

Is there a movement to the pain? Does the pain move in a certain direction? Is the pain pulsating, throbbing or constant?

What emotions are present when you think of the pain?

Write down all of the answers, using your client's own words.

Verify his description, for example: Client says, "feels like there is a knife stuck in my back"...You respond "the pain feels like there is a knife stuck in your back?"

Once you have exhausted every detail about the description, it is time to create change. For example:

- A knife can be pulled out
- A fire can be doused with water
- A square object can be rounded off
- A color can be changed by infusing light
- A rotation can change direction
- A shooting pain can be sent the other way
- A throbbing pain can be dulled by pouring jelly on it
- A pulsating pain can be put on a timer
- A taste can be changed by biting into a lemon
- A sound can be changed by turning it down like a radio
- A feeling can be changed by infusing love (the love from a pet, self love, universal love or a special person)

And now that you have completed this very simple exercise, thank your body once again for doing the very best to keep you informed about what is going on.

Taking in another deep breath, I would like you to focus once again on the muscles around the area of discomfort and allow all them to relax even more...as you focus on (*insert area of pain*) tell me on a scale of 0 – 10...what the level of discomfort is right now.

Continue building expectation that in the days to come this level of comfort will increase...

Emerge client

Cancer Companion

by Helen Bremner

This is designed to help cancer clients RELAX even more deeply, and provide some control over symptoms and worries, helping them cope better...to be happier and healthier. It will complement any medical treatments that are being provided. Use specific portions of it according to your client's needs. Following induction:

We begin our journey in a wonderful, safe, and beautiful cave. Here, you feel calm, just by being here...The more you relax, the more beautiful things you see...amazing crystals that scatter shafts of coloured light across the cave floor...sunlight that shines down from a hole in the cave roof...You notice a beanstalk, climbing up from where it was planted on the cave floor, reaching towards the light...it is always here...whether you are here or not...whether thousands of people are staring at it, or not...it continues to strive...true to itself...Making changes that suit it...Growing in a new direction because that is what is good for it...

You know, that one day, this pale yellowish, sickly beanstalk is going to reach the hole in the cave roof. You know that it will reach the sunlight, and become green and strong. You will visit this cave regularly, noticing how well the beanstalk is growing; how it gets closer, and closer and closer...every single day, until that momentous day when all the struggling is over, and the beanstalk has reached the sunlight outside...and it gets healthier and healthier every day...blossoming and blooming in the glory of its new life...

There is a well at the centre of the cave. Move towards it. Know that drinking from this well connects you with two essential parts of your being...two parts which are essential for good health and happiness: your inner healer and your inner hero. Your inner healer is that part which mends your finger when you cut it...you don't need to think about what blood cells to send where, and how to make new skin, it *just happens* when the inner healer takes over...until one day, you forget to remember and remember to forget that you ever cut your finger...and the same can go for all sorts of things that need healing...and strengthening...Ask your inner healer to take over, and to work as well on every single part of you as it has done for you the times it magically healed your finger... Send it to the parts that need it the most first...

The other part is your inner hero: that superhuman part of you that has got you through those times which were so difficult that you had no clue how you made it through...that part, always walking 2 to 3 steps ahead of you, clearing the path for you, making things just a little bit easier...Your inner healer can protect you from any further pain or damage... Ask it to take over, and to allow you to rest...Drinking from this well connects you strongly to these parts of your inner being.

Take the cup from the side of the well. It's your cup, just for you...and drink the cool healing water...recharge those batteries; feel stronger, calmer, happier, healthier and more in control...And when you've drunk enough, and you feel 10 times more strong, 10 times more calm, happy and in control of every thought, every feeling, every physical and mental experience, you can put your cup down, knowing that you can return here whenever you wish, simply by imagining yourself back in the wonderful cave, or by sipping from a glass of cool water in the waking state...

When you've done that, *you are ready* to walk across the cave floor to a wonderful, safe staircase, which leads to the basement of relaxation...to your perfect place. And in a moment, we're going to go down that staircase...

Make your way now to the 10 steps which make up that stairway...that safe stairway to relaxation...

Neatly carved into each step are the words 'relax even more'...Also carved are the words 'I am calm, relaxed and in control of my thoughts, my feelings and all of my body and what I experience'...

To your left is a large trunk...It can hold anything and everything that you ever want to put in there. There's ALWAYS room for more...I want you to put into that trunk everything that ever bothered you: your worries, your anxieties, your pains...people who have scared or hurt you, events which caused you damage...People who've let you down...Throw them in! Illnesses, diseases, cruel and unfair life events...everything unpleasant that you can think of...just pile it all in...put in your worries, anxieties, relationships, stresses at work...things that people have said or done that have caused you distress or humiliation...times when people let you down...times when you ran out of energy to keep fighting...any feelings of guilt, anxiety, unworthiness...throw them all in. Just like taking off a huge, wet, heavy fur coat with thousands of pockets containing all the things that ever bothered you, ever made you feel angry or sad...take a break from carrying all those worries with you...and *let them go*...

Throw in all those things which have held you back from being the best you that you can be...The true you...Offload

374

procrastination...then close the lid, draw the bolt, and lock the padlock that only you have the key to, and leave the trunk where it lies, to one side at the top of the stairs...this trunk will be here when you come back- you can then take back any of the problems which you want to keep with you...or you can *choose* to *leave them behind*, at the top of the stairs...it's your choice...

So, for now, just leave the trunk at the top of the stairs... I'm going to count you down from 10 to 1...with each step, you are ten times as relaxed as you were the step before, becoming more and more relaxed with every step you take, every breath you breathe, every word that I say and every thought that you think...Recognising the important role that being relaxed has on improving your immune system, on helping you to fight invaders...to fight the baddies!

You relax more with every step down, with every decreasing number...when you reach the number 1, you arrive at the basement of relaxation. It's your perfect place: perfect because you make it that way. It can be somewhere real, or imagined... or somewhere in between...It can be some excellent quality 'me' time, or you can have someone special, or several people who are special with you...You can reconnect with people who have passed away by using your imagination to think about what they would say to help you if they could talk to you now... The choice is yours...It's ALWAYS your choice...When you reach your perfect place, you automatically will be SOO relaxed, so calm and know you are so safe...Drifting down into the deepest, most relaxed state you've ever been in...Continuing your healing journey...Going even deeper today than you've ever gone...to make the changes at a fundamental level within your body and your mind...to work with whatever medical treatments you have...to enhance their success, to become one amazing entity for miraculous healing...

Notice that *every* step has the words 'relax even more' carved neatly into it...Also carved are the words 'I am calm, relaxed and in control of my thoughts, my feelings and all of my body and all that I experience'...and notice that you *want* to relax more with every passing second...with every slow and comfy breath that you take, with every word that I say, and with every thought that you think. YOU GO DEEPER.

(*Use staircase deepening, counting down from 10 to 1*)

And...1...Reaching your perfect place. It's perfect because you make it that way. Everything is *exactly* the way you want it. Your perfect place is perfect for you. It can be the same, reassuring, wonderful place every time you visit it, or it can be new and exciting every time. The choice is always yours. You can choose your company, or you can have some good-quality 'me' time. Spend some time now, exploring this magical place, where *you feel fantastic*!

Amplify these fabulous feelings of well-being, health, strength, inner contentment, peace and love... and when they're at their maximum, and you truly feel wonderful, inside and out, I want you to capture these wonderful feelings between a thumb and a forefinger... Make a ring of healing with your thumb and finger... and feel that tingling spreading up your hands, your arms, to your head: creating an explosion of positivity in your brain, knocking away negativity...and the blood in your brain is recycled around the rest of your body...positivity spreads throughout every cell in your body...Every muscle, every organ, is flooded by this positivity, as, like pac-mans, the positive cells engulf and destroy any residual negativity...

Remember that you can feel this good at any time that you choose to do so, merely by making that thumb and finger into the ring of healing...and allowing the amazing feelings to automatically get stronger and stronger...Connect to that inner healer even more strongly now...And now, allow your hands to relax back into a more comfortable position, as you realise just how much progress you've made, and you are so proud of yourself for all the work you've put in, and how much better your life is becoming, day by day (by day)...

As you look up, you notice a beautiful bubble falling down towards you from way up above. It gets larger and larger, the closer it gets to you...larger and larger...larger and larger...closer and closer...until it reaches you on the ground. It's large enough for you to step inside, and you do so...breathing in the clear, cool, healthy air...protected...safe. Everything negative drains out of the bubble, as you are surrounded by all the positive things in your life...thoughts, deeds, wonderful memories...Like a magnet, the bubble attracts wonderful, positive things to you...and pushes away negative things...Things people do and say that are kind, and that are helpful to you, reach you and add to the happiness inside your bubble. Things people do and say that are unkind or pointless just bounce off the bubble back at them: you remain entirely surrounded by calm, happy, healthy thoughts. Continue to wear this bubble force field as your brightly-coloured suit of armour that protects you.

You have the strength to achieve the level of calm and comfort that you want...be gentle with yourself...be kind...treat yourself like the best friend that you need and deserve, instead of the worst enemy that you have been at times, and it will be easy...Hear the voice of someone who loves you unconditionally...let it be their voice, their words which you use to talk to yourself with. Encourage yourself when things don't go as well as they might... and praise yourself *SO* much when you achieve what you set out to do. Give yourself the encouragement you need...

Let go of all old, useless ideas and symptoms of a struggle from the past...and let these go forever...allow them to just drift away...drift away, making space for a better, happier, healthier life...where you are in control of everything that you experience...as you can bring every single aspect of your life under your *control* now...

Thoughts become things...What the mind can conceive, the mind can achieve... Recognise that you have already made so many wonderful changes that have had a positive impact on your life...Know the power of your own thoughts...Imagine how wonderful life will be once you've closed this chapter...and begin to create it now...and choose to make more changes, and have bigger achievements...

Now, your guardian angel comes to watch over you with a healing and loving gaze...Just being near you is enough for you to receive their loving, healing touch...I want you to leave your body behind, safe, in your perfect place...Every 1 second of real time is equivalent to an hour of real time, spent healing and being at peace, in total comfort at the mind spa...You've already been in your perfect place for several minutes...That's several times 60 hours of healing, forgiveness and peace you've received...

Let your mind now drift and float free from your body...find yourself in a corridor of doors...one of which in particular draws you to it...One door that seems to be somehow calling you to it...more so than the others. Make your way to the door, and understand that this door leads to a *good* place, where you can make the changes that you wish to make...and you may be delighted at how easy it is to make these changes...and just how wonderfully the changes last for you...

Open the door, and go into the room in front of you. It is safe here...you are safe here. Safe to explore...You are in the boiler room. This room is full of control panels...All of them are very simple. Each dial goes from zero...the minimum...to 10, the absolute maximum...There is a control panel for every emotion, every experience you'll ever have...

In front of you is the control panel for relaxation...zero is not relaxed at all, perhaps stressed, and 10 is *the most relaxed you could ever* imagine anyone *be*-ing...Tell me, what number is your relaxation at right now? 0 is not at all...and 10 is the most relaxed you could ever imagine anyone being...What number is your relaxation at right now? And what number would you like it to be? If your number is anything less than 10, what number would someone who loves you unconditionally like it to be? What would I want for you? Yes, I want you to have your relaxation at 10...so just turn it up... Turn the dial to 10, and notice all the wonderful feelings of being completely relaxed, calm and comfortable come flooding through every part of your body. Feel your shoulders go back, released from tension, feel yourself drifting as you are freed...Enjoy every detail that makes the difference between not being relaxed, and being completely relaxed...And lock the dial into position using the PIN number that only the most positive part of your mind has access to.

There's another panel next to the one for relaxation. This one is for your ability to heal... 0 is the least: not at all able to actively heal...and ten is the most wonderful ability to re-grow, to renew and to become stronger than you've ever been...What number is your ability to heal at right now?... And what number do you want it to be? Make sure that you really do want it to be at ten, and turn it up...Right up to 10...Notice all the differences between where you were, and how good it feels now...And lock the dial into position using the PIN number that only the most positive part of your mind has access to.

There's a panel here for feeling sick...Feeling sick is useful if you've over-eaten, or drunk too much...but in treatment, it's useless...It just distracts you from your important focus of getting better... So I want you to recognise that this panel needs always to be as low as possible. You know that you CAN control feelings so well, that you CAN turn a feeling of nausea off completely...or you can have a low number such as 1 or 2...Practise turning the dial down, turning it down to 0...So that if nausea begins to get your attention, you can turn that dial *so* easily to 0, and get on with your important job of healing...of augmenting the treatment you're receiving...And lock the dial into position using the PIN number that only the most positive part of your mind has access to.

There's also a panel for pain. Zero is no pain at all, total comfort...And 10 is the worst pain you could ever imagine anyone having to endure... Notice where your And 10 is the worst pain you could ever imagine anyone having to endure...Notice where your dial is right now... And if it's less than 10, I want you to do something a little strange: turn it right up very briefly...and when you're at 10, turn it swiftly right back to 0...and really enjoy feeling right back where you want it to be. And lock the dial into position using the PIN number that only the most positive part of your mind has access to. You **choose** what you experience. You created pain that you didn't have...and you got rid of pain that you did have...Practise this...so if your pain ever does get to a level which is greater than you want it to be, you can control it easily...just by imagining turning the dial to where you do want it to be...Experience natural, total comfort as you filter out of your experience and awareness any sensations which you can do better without...

What an amazing tool the mind is! Now imagine all the possibilities that having such a wonderful mind can bring you! And know that thoughts become things...Well done, you!

Know that you can do this whenever you want or need to, in the waking state, just by imagining yourself back in this room, or just visualising a control panel ahead of you... Easily and ably, **you can do this**...

You know **you are good enough**. You believe in yourself. You feel comfy, calm, safe and relaxed...with every part of your body and mind...that one glorious whole.

Remember the pain control panel...remember that I asked you to turn your pain right up to the maximum...and then right down to nothing...remember how you created pain that you didn't have AND you got rid of pain that you did have. Your imagination is amazing: use this talent to help yourself so much more.

There may be times in the waking state, when the dials are not exactly as you would wish them to be...Practise turning them to the best positions, and locking them into place. Enjoy the immediate and amazing, complete relief as everything becomes exactly the way you want it to be, just by turning a dial. Remember to use this for yourself in the waking state whenever you wish to, or need to have immediate changes happening for your benefit.

Each morning when you awake, from this moment forward, you awaken with an inner warm glow of confidence, a renewed optimism for life, and a more positive attitude towards doing whatever it is that you want for yourself in your next step...Every day in every way, your life is becoming better and better, and sooo much easier...

Leaving the boiler room, now, go back out to the corridor of doors...Another door is drawing you to it...just as the boiler room one did before...You open the door, and find that it leads to a beautiful walled garden...only you have the key to your garden...Go towards the door and unlock it. People can only come here with an invitation from you... Go into your beautiful garden, where it is always somewhere between early spring and summer...never too hot, never too cold, and experience those wonderful feelings of calm, relaxation, comfort and control over every thought, every feeling...notice how they increase...just by spending time here in your garden. Feeding, weeding, watering and nourishing the garden of your dreams...

In the centre of the garden is a huge oak tree, which was planted as a tiny acorn on the day that you were born. This oak tree is strong...Yet the leaves and smaller branches above you bend and flex with the breezes...Learn what you need to from the tree, which would have snapped and died in the first storm that came along, if it hadn't bent and flexed with the breezes...and because it was flexible, this enormous, wonderful, healthy tree stands in front of you today. Move past beautiful flowers and plants to the flower beds...There is a flower bed here...once there were beautiful flowers and plants here...

Today, an enormous weed is strangling the other flowers and plants...choking them...depriving them of food and water...You wonder what could have happened to this flower bed...and you notice that there's a name plaque...you rub away years of dust and dirt to reveal what's written on the plaque...It says (name's) dreams'...This flower bed is your old dreams which you planted a long time ago...With a great sense of indignation, you pull at that weed with determination...and to your surprise, it comes away easily...shrivels up...and turns to dust...blowing away on the gentle breeze...You look back at the bed, and notice that the plants and flowers are already beginning to recover...You water them and feed them carefully...and they begin to thrive...You notice what those dreams are...Dreams about thriving...being strong, happy, and healthy...Know that should any weeds crawl back and start to take hold of your dreams again, that they will come away easily in your hand...and turn to dust, blowing away on the gentle breeze.

Next to the flower bed of your old dreams is a freshly-dug bed...You realise that some of the dreams you planted a long time ago are no longer relevant to your life...It's ok to let them fade...But here, a new bed is dug, ready for you to plant your new dreams...Things that you want for yourself right now...That freedom, perhaps...Health now meaning something more profound to you than perhaps it once did...Plant the bulbs, plants, flowers and seeds of your new dreams...Water them, feed them...Return to your garden

383

regularly to nurture them...Some dreams can be a wonderful surprise to you later... Something you don't consciously realise that you want has been planted by your unconscious mind...Place the shiny new plaque with pride. Survey all you've achieved, and be so proud of yourself. Recognise that there's achievements that you've made that, at one time, you didn't think were possible. You ARE amazing! And you CAN do anything you choose to.

Notice how well your plants and flowers are doing in the bed of your old dreams. Look how much they've grown, in the short time you've been here...

Remember to feed, weed and water them regularly. Visit your garden whenever you wish to have a top-up of feeling good, or you want to feel better in times of challenge.

Colorectal Cancer Surgery Specific:

There's a stream which magically appears at one end of the garden through the wall, crosses the garden, and magically disappears through another wall. Move across to the stream now. Visit the upper end of the stream, and put in sticks, twigs, stones, rocks and boulders...make the flow exactly the right pace and speed for you...

Control the flow as it slowly and predictably fills the pond at the other end... And realise that you can wander away, and you will be gently reminded once the pond becomes nearly full...and at this point, you can choose when to return to the pond, reach into it, and pull the plug...Allowing the pond to gently and predictably empty, at just the right time, speed and pace for you...Put the plug back in...And allow it to

384

gently and predictably re-fill... and repeat the procedure as many times a day as it suits you to... it may be enough to do this once...

The pond has been neglected...It needs a landscaper to come and make it work effectively again...The grass around the pond has turned brown...The pond is furred up...The landscaper comes, and cuts away bits of damaged pond...Creating a new route for the stream...At first, this seemed like a scary thing to do...But notice now, how wonderful the new pond is...The landscaper has done an excellent job...and the grass grows back, luscious and green...

Make sure that everything in your garden is exactly the way you want it to be. Pledge to return here very soon, to top up your feelings of well-being, pride in yourself and strength...

Go through the garden door, and lock it behind you.

Return back to the corridor of doors, where another door is grabbing your attention... This seems urgent...and you respond to the door's calling...and you go inside...This room contains a wonderful, living wall...This wall is not a thing of beauty, but it's an amazing, protecting, life-sustaining wall...The wall is becoming weak...You remember how the weed in your garden was strangling your dreams...There's a different sort of weed attacking this wall...It's stuck its roots right into the wall and is taking away its energy and nutrients...It is a form of parasite...It will never stop by choice...It doesn't realise that by draining its host, it will end up killing itself too...

You recognise the parasitic weed for what it is...And you resolve to treat the weed the same way...and to save the wall...By isolating the part of the wall where the weed is infiltrating and infecting the wall, you can starve the weed of its energy and nutrients...

I want you to imagine reducing the flow of energy and nutrients to that weed...that cancer...divert your blood flow away from the weed that's draining from you...Clearly imagine and focus on sending your blood elsewhere, and picture the cancer struggling to survive...its progress stopped...Imagine this in microscopic detail...Send fighting white cells to kill it off...Reduce the blood flow to that area to a trickle...and then turn it off completely...

Back-up arrives and professional wall-protectors move in and take over the main work...But **your** work is the most important...Only you can stop this...Continue to divert the blood flow well away from the weed...and feel the energy returning to your body as the nutrients are used to nurture your body...

Visit this room regularly...Help the team to protect the wall...

Chemotherapy-Specific:

Return now, to the corridor of doors, where yet another door is calling you towards it...

You open the door, and find yourself on a path which leads to a beautiful house...like a stately home...There are lots of rooms...but as you get closer to the dramatic building, you notice that it's in a very bad state...a poor state of repair...You find bits of plasterwork which have amazing intricate details on...You wipe away years of dust and dirt from the floor and walls, you can see that this house is a wonderful place...You decide to clean it up...and return it to its former glory. It takes a lot of energy and effort, and strong cleaning chemicals...but it's WELL WORTH it. To return this beautiful house to its former beauty and amazing strength...and when you have spent hours and hours cleaning every single room, every single door, floor, ceiling and wall...window and decorative mantel piece, you are proud of your work, and your restoration of a national treasure.

Colorectal Specific:

After all that cleaning with strong, toxic chemicals, there is just one more thing which needs doing to renovate this house completely...The drain needs replacing. It's broken...You spend time and energy creating a new drain...a new mechanism. You take advice from specialist plumbers and drain experts. You KNOW how much better it's going to be than the old one. This one will be so easy to use, and you've got the engineers on call to help you to keep it working well and getting rid of all your rubbish. It takes a lot of effort, but you HAVE the energy, and you have the determination to see this project through, because you know the end result is going to be spectacular.

Returning to the corridor, once more...Realising just how much relaxation and healing your body is getting in your perfect place as your mind explores the many exciting rooms that lead from this corridor...You are drawn to another door...

Inside the room there is a baby...A tiny, beautiful baby ...naturally learning to grow and heal...sleeping beautifully

...peacefully...Knowing that it's best to sleep and relax through tough times...And there's an older child, and an old person...They look at you with amazement. They want to know how you have achieved all that you have done in your life...They want to be like you when they grow up. They admire your strength and independence...These are great characteristics, and have already helped you so much in your life...More and more people and children come forward to you, each telling you what it is about you that they admire...It's quite a powerful experience to realise just the unique set of skills and attributes that you have...and these are what will get you through some tough times in your life...

That older person comes up to you now...not sure how old they are, but they're much older than you are now...They say 'thank you, (name). Thank you for all you did...all you went through...your bravery and strength. Because of you, I have lived a long and happy life. I achieved things that I would never have done if you hadn't helped me so much. I'm not sure, but perhaps because of, rather than in spite of, the cancer I once had, my life has become so much more rewarding and special...and it's because of you. Thank you. All the people in this room move towards you in a gentle, supportive group hug...like a set of Russian dolls...

You realise that every single one of them is you...From the baby, all the way up to the old person...All the (name)s that ever were, and all the (name)s that ever will be, are in this one room...ready to help you with that unique set of skills and qualities... And you can return here at any time that life challenges you, and you have doubts...and you will be reassured about your future, and refocused on adding to your achievements and skills...

Leave the room, and return to the corridor...

In the corridor, there is a strange grub...it's crawling towards a dark corner...Tired, and exhausted...When it reaches the corner, you watch with fascination as it begins to spin a silky weave...That tired, fed up little creature covers itself with its weave, continuing to spin the silky thread until all of it is protected by its cocoon...You know a better place for this little grub to stay...So you gently take the cocoon to your perfect place, setting it down in a safe place, where there will be plenty for it to eat if it gets hungry...Think now, about what your cocoon will be made of...What support you will need, who you wish to have by your side...

Begin to make your own cocoon now...adding to it as necessary...climb inside...work like you've never worked before, seeking help from your inner hero...from your inner healer...Practise controlling symptoms and expressing emotions...spend time in your garden...clean that house...make use of your Russian dolls...your healing anchors (which have been set up previously), and keep your guardian angel with you at all times as you wear your protective bubble.

And whilst you are practising these protective, healing, helpful techniques, and becoming stronger...the grub in the cocoon that you saved is also growing...it's getting stronger too, day by day...you are protected in your cocoon...your inner hero taking over for you at times of challenge, allowing you to rest...your inner healer working in harmony with your wish to create a better life for yourself...You know that when these days of challenge have passed...the creature in the cocoon will begin to stir...and your cocoon will have served its purpose...the grub will have become the most amazing butterfly that you've ever seen...having changed so dramatically and having become something way beyond our understanding of the ability to cope and create positive changes...seeing insects, caterpillars and grubs can remind you of the creature in the cocoon...can remind you of your own cocoon, until you are ready to stretch your new wings, and start your new life as magical and as different as that beautiful BUTTERFLY!...and whenever you see a butterfly, you can have a gentle reminder that hope is realistic...

Now it's time we started to make our way back...

Move back to the stairway, feeling stronger, healthier, and calmer...More sure of a positive future...Notice now, that the words on the stairs have changed...They are a private, positive message to you...

At the top of the stairs is your trunk... with those stresses and worries in, you can open it if you want...or you can **choose to leave them behind**, in the past...Feel good, feel strong, and feel happier...without that baggage...

And in a moment, I'm going to count you back up those stairs...when you get to the 10th stair, you will be wide awake, feeling good, feeling relaxed, feeling calm and happy...bringing with you all you have learned today, adding to it every single day...

1...Everything I have suggested remaining with you and growing stronger in every way.
2...Your mind and your body now joining back together to become one glorious whole... all parts working together to achieve your goal of excellent health...
3...Realizing now how much influence you have on how you feel... and that you choose to feel calm, comfortable, relaxed and in control...

4...Calling on your inner healer and your inner hero every day to make life's challenges easier for you.

5...Knowing that your large reservoir of strength, will power, and self-esteem is growing, day by day, and increasing as a reflex action that you don't even need to <u>think about</u> .
6...Lighter and brighter...
7...8...More aware of the room around you...
9...On my next count, your eyes will open, and you'll be wide awake... feeling calmer, more relaxed, with your immune system activated...
And 10...Open your eyes, feeling calm and positive.

Non-Smoker

by Joanna Cameron

1) Cigarettes are not physically addictive. Drinking water (dehydration) and eating fruit (replaces the desire for sugar which is in cigarettes) help. Bottom line - I have never seen anyone who lied, cheated, stole and ended up in jail for smoking addiction.

2) Cigarettes are not mentally addictive. What the person needs is oxygen and deep breathing covers that!

3) Cigarettes are not your friend - does a friend stab you in the back?!

Do not use this process unless you know that your client acknowledges that he/she is ready to become a nonsmoker and is motivated on a level of 10 out of 10. (EFT tapping is a great way to increase motivation prior to induction.)

Now, please get in a position where you would have the most comfort. That's right. And make sure that you have turned off your cell phone and other noise devices. This is a signal to your unconscious mind that you will give the suggestions your full attention. Just find a spot that you can focus your eyes on and take a big breath...IN...OUT...And again. Breathe IN...OUT...Now close your eyes.

Imagine that there is a white light coming in through your forehead and the white light is going to progressively relax every nerve, muscle, and fiber of your body...leaving you totally relaxed. As you think about the muscles of your forehead...smooth and relaxed, they do relax. And the white light moves into the muscles of your eyes, relaxing your eyes, and into the muscles of your face and your jaw. The jaw is a place where stress and tension gather, so if you wish to open your mouth just a little bit and relax your jaw...that is fine. And the white light moves into the muscles of your neck, relaxing your neck, and into the muscles of your shoulders. And now you breathe in and as you breathe out, you relax all the muscles of your chest. With every breath you take, you become more and more relaxed. And the sound of my voice relaxes you. You can let go of any other sounds...these are unimportant.

The white light moves down your arms, relaxing all the muscles, and into your hands. You may have warmth in the palms of your hands and you may have tingling in your fingertips...that is perfectly fine. And you may feel that you could barely lift your arms...they are so heavy, so heavy, so relaxed. And now you breathe in again and as you breathe out, you relax all the muscles of your legs, all the way down to your toes. You are now perfectly relaxed.

As you are sitting there, taking a few relaxing deep breaths, it is a good thing to wonder how your conscious mind may wander or drift or your conscious mind may become aware of how the chair feels beneath your legs, a sound in your environment or even your own breathing. And your conscious mind can forget those things that your unconscious mind may remember. And you can just allow yourself the luxury of deeper state of light trance or a lighter state of deep trance. And your unconscious mind can remember to forget those things or forget to remember those things which your conscious mind remembers. That's right. Because there is nowhere to go right now but know where you are going...you are going to a nonsmoking place.

Now, imagine a peaceful and special place. This could be the beach or the mountains by a stream, or a garden with a seat...any place is perfectly fine. And there is a staircase with ten steps, leading you to your peaceful and special place. And with every step you go down on the staircase, you double your relaxation. Beginning at the tenth step now - you take a careful step down, going deeper and deeper. 9, 8, 7, 6, 5, 4— nearly there—3, 2, 1.

You are now in your peaceful and special place and maybe you can even feel it. You are alone there and there is no one to disturb you. And every time that you go to this place in your mind, you intuitively know that you can let go of the stresses and tensions of everyday life. They can just bounce off and away from you, like water off a duck's back. You have a sense of well-being, tranquility, and peacefulness.

And with every breath you take, you become more and more peaceful and my voice will go with you as we take this journey of change. And the sound of my voice will relax you more and more.

Think about your eyes. Your eyes have become so relaxed that they are one piece of skin. In a moment, I will count from 1 to 3 and ask you to try in vain to open your eyes. Your eyes are stuck, stuck like glue and this is perfectly fine. The more that you try to open them, the more that they are stuck. You may find that you can move the muscles of your eyebrows, but your eyes are stuck together. Okay, 1, 2, 3—try to open your eyes, try harder to open your eyes. Okay, forget about your eyes now and go deeper into hypnosis.

And now your legs are just like concrete, they are stuck to the floor... In a moment I am going to ask you to try, try in vain to move your legs but you will not be able to do so as your legs are like concrete – they are stuck to the floor. I am going to count from one to three and your legs are unstuck. 1, 2, Free! And now I am going to count from one to three and you will open your eyes. I will then say sleep and snap my fingers and you will go into a trance, ten times deeper. 1, 2, 3, opening up your eyes. Snap. And again, one two three, snap. Sleep now.

In the future whenever I say the word sleep, you will be go into a very deeper state of trance. And every time you go into a trance, you will experience the state more perfectly, deeply and completely than the last.

Your mind has now become so open to everything that I say and everything that I say will have an ever increasing effect over the way that you think and feel.

Today is the day that you are a non-smoker. Today is the first day of your nonsmoking life. That's right. You have made this decision for all the right reasons and you are so motivated to let go of the habit. Because you realize that you have given up an unhealthy habit that can easily be replaced by a healthy habit...like drinking lots of water. You are gaining health and losing an enemy. And just as you have been successful in so many endeavors...then you will be successful at this but you are the person NOW that you said that you always wanted to be...a nonsmoker.

You are a nonsmoker. From now on...the thought of smoking a cigarette will be disgusting to you. You denounce the habit. You understand that smoking impeded not you're your breathing but your ability to relax and it never increased your self esteem and contributed to boredom. Enough! Your last cigarette was a symbol of that. You have had enough of dirt in your system. In fact, the smell of smoke will be disgusting to you... positively revolting! Imagine throwing a pack of cigarettes into the trash. You have had it. You want cigarettes off and away from you. So you will go home today and clean every last speck of smoking from your life. Wash out any clothes. It feels so good to just clean and get rid of this habit once and for all...because YOU ARE A NONSMOKER, A NONSMOKER.

I wonder...and it is a good thing to wonder...if you know that the main ingredient in cigarette smoke is methane gas. And, of course, methane gas mostly comes from would you believe...cow farts! Cow farts! That's right...cows pass a lot of gas. Just imagine yourself now lifting the tail of that cow and breathing in. Go on...take a crack at it. Maybe it is a little bit wet...I don't know about you but I would want to **PASS** on that... would not want to be the **BUTT** of that joke. How good it feels to just pass on that cigarette.

Let's get a new picture. Imagine yourself in a meadow of spring flowers...hyacinths, primroses, bluebells, daffodils...all those flowers that you love. It is a picture perfect day, bright and clear and you feel great. In the distance you see an old fashioned English castle with a moat and masses of water around it. Being a curious person, you decide to explore. You walk to the castle and open the door. It creaks. Inside it is all dark. But there is light shining in through a turret. And in that band of light...you see dirt. However, there is a spigot and a scrubbing brush so you start to work. Scrubbing all the dirt of the walls and watching it being washed away down the drain. You keep going until it is all clean. And it takes lots and lots of water. And when you have finished cleaning you go back out again to the meadow. You are amazed that all your senses have opened up. You can feel the fresh air on your skin. And the SMELL of the flowers...ooh, the fresh smell of hyacinths. You feel proud of yourself...the work that you have done. So you lie down and you take a nap.

And when you wake up tomorrow it will the first full day of your nonsmoking life. You feel great. You made the right decision for all the right reason and you carried it thru and you feel fantastic. Imagine yourself going through your day without a cigarette. You feel great. There is a smile on your face.

And you continue to drink lots of water and with every breath you take you become more confident in your ability to set a goal and carry it through. You are a nonsmoker...a nonsmoker. You imagine yourself a year from today. You did it. And it was easy and effortless. It took a motivated decision. And you think of the money that you have saved over the last year and you give yourself a special treat on that day. Because YOU are the center of your universe. YOU ROCK.

And when you sit down at the dinner table you eat the right foods in the right proportions. You really like fruits and vegetables. When you go to the store you are really attracted to the produce department all the colorful, freshly misted vegetables. And you eat slowly and really enjoy your food. But you eat the correct amount for you and when you have finished eating, you push away from the table and stop eating. You refrain from eating processed food and sugar. You know that these foods are bad for you and your emotions. You want to be healthy in all aspects of your life. You take up a program of exercise and imagine yourself doing this...maybe you like to take a walk outside or go to the gym. Every day in every way you are becoming healthier and happier.

Now, I want you to make your arm into a bar of steel. Stiff and rigid. Stiff and rigid. A bar of steel. Your arm lifts out of your lap and is a bar of steel. Imagine that I am pushing down on that arm now. But your arm rises up as I push down, as it is a bar of steel. Your arm is your unconscious mind. You will only be able to return the arm to your lap when you are totally satisfied with your decision. You are a nonsmoker, a nonsmoker. You are a nonsmoker, a nonsmoker. You have made the decision for all the right reasons. You desire to breathe deeply and breathe healthy air. Breathing in deeply now.

And you now imagine that healing white light, healing every nerve, muscle cell and fiber of your body. Cleansing and healing all of your body. And now imagine that white light coming out of your body and into the bodies of those closest to you...cleansing and healing. So now you are ALL the light.

You remember this feeling of the white light and being a non-smoker. You want to be in the light. You want to be healthy. You are a non-smoker. And with every breath, you take your body heals itself.

So anytime that you put your head on the pillow and your intention is sleep...you will be the world's best sleeper and will sleep thru the night and will get up in the morning... feeling relaxed, refreshed, feeling fantastic and the first thing that you will say either out loud or to yourself, "I am a non-smoker!"

I am going to count from one to five and you will come back in the room twenty per cent with each count...remembering whenever I say SLEEP...that you will fall back into hypnotic trance. One, coming up, two feeling great, three you are a nonsmoker, four stretching five eyes wide open. Welcome back!! And thank you for including me in your decision and process to stop smoking. May I be the first to congratulate you! Congratulations!

Smoking Cessation Tiger Story

by Marion Robb

This is a script that I use as part of my smoking cessation protocols. I primarily use parts-based hypnotherapy for smoking cessation, but developed this script particularly for a young woman who wished to cease smoking to have children. I had previously, using parts therapy, helped her cut down significantly, however, upon using this script, she left beaming, and six months post-treatment was still a non-smoker.

Once upon a time there was a little girl who lived near a dense jungle in a hot, dusty country. Everything smelt hot, the earth, the trees, the grass, and even the little girl's skin and hair, smelt all day of the sunshine and heat. And so it was that when the women returned to the village with the water, everyone came to sit and talk and sup some water, all the people, all the birds, all the dogs and all the animals, came to relax in the middle of the village and have a long cool drink and cool down. And then the village would congregate beside the cooking pot and eat the good things which the adults had caught for them to eat that day, and life was simple and clean and good.

All day long for years and years the little girl stayed safe and sound near her friends and family in her little hut in the village and didn't stray away from the path. And she grew healthy and bonny but the heat was a constant source of irritation to her and she longed to be cool. The heat made her skin prickle and the birds squawk, and the dogs lie still and boring under the shady tree.

And sometimes the little girl would say to her Daddy, "Daddy can I go and play in the jungle?" and Daddy would say "No, Dear Heart, the jungle is a dangerous place, where dark things live and may swallow you up. It is more enjoyable to stay here with your family and friends – we will take care of you. It is difficult sometimes not to be cool, but it is better here in the heat than to be lost to the dark. Do venture into the forest path."

But as the girl grew older she grew more and more adventurous and day by day, she ventured closer to the edge of the jungle forest. The jungle looked deep and dense and cool and relaxing. One day, the little girl, put a foot off the path, and stepped, for the very first time, into the deep, dark jungle. And at first, she wasn't very sure whether she actually liked it – in many ways it didn't feel right, it didn't feel natural, the smells and the sounds were wrong, as if she were doing the wrong thing in breathing it in. Although the air in the jungle forest was also hot and dusty, something in the air seemed dark and wrong and managed to get down into her very lungs, under her skin, and in her hair. And because it was so dark, her bonny skin got no light, and so the dark and the dustiness settled in her skin and turned her bonny skin a little more grey every day. Everyone knows that if you deny your body sunlight, or breathe in things you should not, you do not look as healthy as you should.

In the jungle undergrowth, things rustled and moved, and all around a sense of danger persisted. But still the little girl disregarded her own instincts and every day she walked a little more into the forest on her own. And as she walked she had to be very careful where she was putting her feet, as roots and branches stuck out of the ground and waited to trip her up, but eventually she became more used to the forest, and so, even though she still knew it wasn't safe for her to be there, every day she stayed in the forest a little bit longer.

There came a day when the rustling in the undergrowth grew louder, and very carefully, the little girl parted the leaves of some bushes, and there in front of her, was a tiger cub, with the most beautiful fiery eyes. The tiger was bright orange like a flame, with dark streaks across its pelt and as the little girl looked at the tiger cub she was entranced and she could not, no matter how she tried, she could not **give up** seeing her tiger cub friend for long.

Each and every day, more and more often, the little girl would go to the forest to play with her tiger cub friend, to feed it, and just be with it, and to let the tiger cub be with her. Soon though, her friends and family began to notice there were scratches and little bites on the girl's arms. "Oh dear," said the little girl's Daddy, "What have you been doing to yourself? Are you being careful?" And the little girl replied, "I've just been playing with my friend...she gets a bit rough sometimes."

"Hmm" said Daddy. "Well, sometimes friends can seem like friends, but deep down, they're not, and those are the sort of friends who can hurt you. So do be careful my little dear and **give up now** going into the forest". And the little girl, thinking suddenly of a tiny little antelope deer, bouncing about the forest in front of her tiger cub friend.

She went into the forest and she said to her friend, "Tiger cub, if you saw a baby antelope, would you chase it?" And her friend said, "Oh, my little dear friend...I am a tiger cub. And every day I grow a little larger, and a little hungrier. So surely, one day I will be strong enough to follow my nature and catch the little deer. And in fact, my dear little friend, one day, we can no longer be friends, as on that day I will finally be stronger than you, no matter how big you grow and how fast you may run, and surely one day, I will **give up** being your friend and be strong enough to follow my nature and catch you!"

And the tiger cub laughed merrily and loudly as if it was a great big joke, and the little girl, laughed, too, as she didn't believe that the playful, friendly cub would ever grow up into a dangerous tiger. It almost seemed that the more the little girl played with the friend who was no good to her, and the more damage the tiger cub did, and no matter how much the forest air hurt her lungs, and robbed her bonny skin of air, the more the little girl ignored the dangers.

And so, it came to pass one day that the little girl went to see the tiger cub, and the tiger cub was a cub no more, but was now a beautiful, deadly, living flame of a beast that burnt brightly in the dark with a hunger as ferocious as its bite. And the claws of the tiger were a terrible thing to behold, and the teeth of the tiger were sharp and fearsome. And between the claws and teeth of the beautiful tiger cub lie a little antelope deer.

And no matter how the little girl had become a creature of the forest, in her heart of hearts she knew she could not outrun her deadly friend, for that dreaded day had arrived...when her friend turned from a playmate to a tormentor. And she knew it was time **to give up now**.

So as she grew older and wiser and turned from a girl to a woman, she began to approach that tiger more and more cautiously, more and more silently, and less and less often.

It was difficult at first to turn her back on the friend, with whom she had played and spent many hours, but a strange thing happened....

One day she found that she drew a line over the entrance to the forest. She looked at it with a feeling of relief as she knew she would never step over that line again. As she returned to the sunlight and the heat of the village, as she returned to the watering hole and the daily cook-outs, her skin once again bloomed, and her eyes grew larger and moist and she grew as bonny as if she had never put a foot in the forest. And her scars healed and her lungs and her hair got rid of the dank air of the forest.

And eventually the little girl had children of her own and she watched them carefully and every time she heard a tiger roar in the forest, she would shake her head at her children and say "The tiger nearly caught your mother, do not venture into the forest path."

And just like that little girl, you can imagine stepping over that line for the last time and allowing all the foulness that is smoking to just leave your body, as if it all just leaves your body in a smoky, smelly, ashy, brown, sticky foulness, right there on the road, leaving it all behind you now. That's right. And as you imagine yourself crossing over that line you become completely a non-smoker now and you are so glad that you notice a feeling of lightness and relief, that the air smells sweeter, things taste better and brighter. That the air that goes down into your lungs is pure and healthy now, that's right, that you are no longer a slave to nicotine, that you really are a non-smoker. And you say to yourself:

I am a non-smoker...nothing will make me want to hurt

myself or my children in that way again.

I AM a non-smoker and nothing will make me want to hurt myself or my children in that way again, that's right.

(*Repeat with different emphasis*)

I have no desire to taste smoke again...I have no desire to set fire to a nasty-flavored stick and put it in my mouth again...I have no desire to hurt my health by smoking...I am a non-smoker...

And now I am going to count to 10 and when I reach 10 you will be back in the room, you will feel alert, and energized and happy to be a non-smoker.

You will forget to remember or remember to forget what it was like to be a smoker and all that smoking will leave you with now is a vague sense of distaste, that's right

Ready...1,2,3,4,5...

Chapter 14 Final Touches

The Roller Coaster Technique

by Iantha Greer

Every once in a while, I get a client who is nervous about 'going under' in a hypnotherapy session. This fear of the unknown can interfere with the hypnotic state, not to mention their ability to relax!

For these clients I have used a mental 'roller coaster' to introduce them to the spectrum of awareness their mind can experience. By going up and down to varying degrees, the client can become comfortable with their own ability to relax and energize. The client travels between a high energy state where they are hyper-aware of their surroundings, and a low energy state where they are only aware of their own consciousness.

This technique works for many reasons:

1. It takes the pressure off. Clients know that even if they cannot relax right away they will have another opportunity.

2. It affirms that they have control over themselves. By moving through these different states of consciousness the client can feel how their thoughts affect their body and mind.

3. It relieves anxiety about losing awareness. Clients know that even if they totally relax, they will become aware again very quickly, so the fear of being 'put under' is removed from the equation.

It is very important to know of any fears or phobias the client has before attempting The Roller Coaster Technique. If there is any fear of roller coasters, heights, etc., it is better to use a train going up over hills and down into valleys, or a yo-yo that slowly goes up and down.

Once you have gone through an initial induction, and the client has begun to relax, you can begin taking them up and down between hyper-awareness and deep relaxation. The duration and frequency depends on the client's needs.

"Now imagine you are on a gentle, slow-moving roller coaster. Ahead of you, in the distance, the track goes up and down, up and down. Some areas of the track are very high, and others are very low. Now you begin to move down, slowly. The track goes down just a little, and you feel slightly more relaxed than before. And you are moving upward now, passing the point of being just awake, and moving into a very energetic state.

The track continues up, and you feel very aware, hyper-aware, of everything around you. You become more and more energized as you travel upward, then the track rounds back toward the ground, and you feel yourself relaxing again. The track goes down much further now. You feel yourself relaxing, deeper, and deeper. Until all you know is you are relaxed and calm. Just as you reach the very bottom of this dip, you become totally relaxed, totally focused inward.

Then you begin to move slowly, gently back up, becoming more aware, more excited. This part of the track goes very, very high. As you continue moving up, you become hyper aware of everything around you, but you are still calm. You may feel as if you are tingling with fast-moving energy, so fast you are vibrating with energy. Just as you reach the top, you feel more awake than you have ever felt.

Then you begin moving down again, gently. Now the track

goes down very, very far, very deep. You feel your body relaxing, your mind focusing inward. Completely relaxed, going deeper and deeper. And it keeps moving down...down... down...Going deeper...and deeper."

I have also had success using this for depression, insomnia, motivation, and increasing energy. It makes a difference in their progress when people realize they can create these feelings of excitement/energy and relaxation/calmness so quickly and effectively.

Talking to Your Body

by Janice Lesley

Use in conjunction with hypnosis or hypnotherapy.

USE your imagination! Play with it! I have been talking to my body for over 20 years in this way and I can guarantee you that this method works in an amazing way, even on the very first try! But of course, practice will make it even easier and more effective for you...

I am always looking for faster and more effective ways to heal and this one fits the bill. Once you get good at it, it can take you under an hour of quick scribbling, reviewing and reducing until you are a left with a sentence that will bring you enlightenment. Once you master this technique you can move on to giving body parts and diseases a bit of personality and begin to dialogue your way out of illnesses. It's all fun, all harmless and all remarkably effective. My kind of "work"!

To start, all you need is a paper and pen and then IMAGINE the area of pain or disease and try to *describe* it (write on paper) what it looks like.... as if you had to DESCRIBE it to someone else!

List some headings that describe your senses, such as Touch, Look, Sound, Taste, Smell...

Then, think about how you might describe it: What is its color, texture, feel, size, etc...and scribble down ALL OF THE ADJECTIVES you can think of on to your paper, under each of your headings (ie: color; red, dark red, like a blood red, a thick, oozy red....)

When you are done and have filled up a sizable portion of your page of paper (!) with adjectives, glance at what you have, and pick the adjectives that stick out the most for you or that have been the most repeated by the use of similar words or ones with similar meanings...(ie: oily, slick, slippery...)

Then do the exercise again using those keys words. For example, say the word 'hard' stuck out the most for you, so do this next: think about what the word "hard" means to you, ie; mean, cold, unapproachable, protective, too protective...

And then quickly review and reduce the list again. After you have done this a few times, you are actually left with just a FEW KEY WORDS, which are a description of your disease or pain and will help you to know it better and why you have it.

Congratulations, you have just successfully dived into the womb of your mind! You avoided the direct and ineffective old way of coping (which clearly wasn't working anymore) and you have discovered another way into your own deeper mind. You have begun to learn a new language based on symbols...a language particular to you and your unconscious mind which will open new pathways for you into self knowledge and, ergo...self healing.

Blessings to you!

Hospice Quilt

Teya Graves

I would like you...to just take a few moments now...to imagine a beautiful...thick... warm...quilt...that is being put together...stitch...by stitch.

Like most quilts ...it's being put together ...by selecting different pieces of material ...and stitching them together. Most pieces... are all the same size...and depending on the design... or the effect you want...you sew one little piece... onto another... as it grows... more...and more meaningful.

Those pieces ...add up to a larger one... and you sew the larger ones together after that. I am not sure...how that makes sense to you...but you can just imagine...each little square...representing a part of your life...and all those little pieces...are made up of your favourite colours...and I wonder...if in one piece...you might see your husband... your marriage...see things that represent your love for him...

And see pieces that represent...his love...and support...for you. And now imagine...stitching pieces...that represent...your Children/Daughter/Son...

Choose bright...beautiful colours...of the softest...most loving materials...and maybe you might even imagine...transferring pictures...onto some of the squares...pictures of happy memories...that you can find in your...deep...subconscious mind now...

...find more...beautiful memories...maybe a child's flower...or first steps...what else do you see? Can you imagine squares...with embroidered names...of people...or places...that made you feel warm...and happy...and loved...and safe.

Create these special pieces now...in the privacy of your own mind...and when you have created...all that you want for now...just raise a finger on one hand so I know...and we will move on.

Wonderful...thank you. You do have many...beautiful pieces...of your life...to stitch together...and if you like...you can continue...to use this visualization...to create more pieces...of the big picture...and the feeling of love...and relaxation.

The only problem...is you can see all those old...dangling threads...that distract from the beauty. See the threads...that represent the things you don't want to be concerned about anymore...so with the intention...of releasing the worries...just cut them off...one at a time.

Find a particularly long thread...that reaches back into your childhood...that represents...an old hurt and just cut it off.

Now find another thread... that just dangles there...thick...and dark...as it represents a worry about _____ (*children/husband/fear of dying, etc.*)

Maybe you see another thread...that's frayed from having too much attention...it looks kind of ugly... because it represents _____ (*or*) something you think about too often...that you can't even change anyway...because it's something from your past... and because it is in the past...it's just a story...that doesn't have any control over you anymore.

(Continue cutting threads that were previously discussed as

negative memories. Use their words as much as possible)

And have one more look...at your beautiful quilt now...with all the pieces...fitting together...to represent the warmth...and the beauty of your life...and the contributions... you have made...to the lives of others...and the contributions...that others have made... to your life.

The old loose threads of the past...have been snipped off...and discarded...so you can focus...on just the love...and the good memories...and the warm feelings now...because your comfort...and your legacy...of the good things of your life...are...what truly matter.

And just imagine now...that you wrap this beautiful quilt around your shoulders... feeling safe...and loved...and accomplished. You know...that when you touch it...you can feel all the love...and caring...that was put into...every stitch.

You have created a masterpiece of art...that is a representation...of your life...and the warmth and love that you created...can be passed on to your husband...and your children...and your grandchildren...as they are...ultimately cloaked...in your love...and your care...

Creating Love and Partnership

by Jagi Egnell

Following induction of your choice:

Feel yourself going deeper and deeper into relaxation...you now understand and appreciate that one of your strongest desires...one of your most cherished wants and needs...is to love and be loved in return...by a companion who will love you unconditionally and passionately forever...You know that for this to occur you must share similar feelings towards each to make that perfect partnership...You notice as your subconscious mind develops a strategy for this to occur by visualizing what you want to attain...your main goal today is to show your subconscious what you want...what you desire in this perfect partnership you are manifesting...

I want you notice that there is writing pad and pencil in front of you...pick up the pencil...and begin to list the qualities you desire in a mate...Notice as you write each quality, you can feel your desire becoming more and more concrete...you know that you are drawing the perfect partner into your life...one who is meant to be with you...I am going to now give you a few moments to write down what you really desire in a perfect partnership....(*pause*)

Now that you have clearly described what you desire in a perfect partnership, imagine yourself now being with this person....you are both happy, relaxed, affectionate...easily sharing emotions and the unconditional love you have for each other...

Visualize and imagine as you both walk hand in hand, looking adoringly into each other's eyes...perhaps you are walking along the sea shore...notice that, each time the water laps over your feet, how your love for each other grows even stronger...Feel the closeness, feel the love between the both of you... (*pause*)

Now you are going to create a special place in your brain to work on creating this perfect partnership...I want you to visualize or imagine seeing a picture of your brain...now notice yourself enlarging this picture...now I want you to find the special part in your brain where you will store qualities you desire in a perfect mate(pause for minute)...notice this part of your brain is created for love with the perfect partner...I want you to take the list you created earlier and store it in this part of your brain(quiet for 1 minute)...now you will notice as you add more qualities you desire in a perfect partnership you will add them to this part of your brain...

I want you to now show your conscious mind where you have stored this information in your subconscious...your conscious mind will find this very quickly...these qualites will radiate from you and the one you truly desire and are meant to be with will be drawn to you...

Now that you a clear picture of what actually want to achieve, you find yourself moving forward instead of backwards....you notice as your confidence in attracting the perfect partnerships increases ten folds...you now know you conscious and subconscious are now working together to draw the perfect mate for you...

You may realize that the relationships you had in past were not with the perfect partner and that is why they did not work out...you can now let go of these relationships and any related hurt to create the perfect partnership you have just created for yourself...

416

You are much stronger for having lived through the hurtful experiences of the past...you know the one who is meant for you is now drawing closer and closer to you...you know that you will recognize each other instantly and know you were meant for each other...

Send out positive affirmations and continue to focus on them to draw the perfect companion for you...You will find yourself repeating after me and sending out positive thoughts and as you do...imagine that your thoughts touch every part of the universe...you know the universe will rearrange itself to provide what you truly desire in a perfect partnership...

Let these affirmations move through your mind now: (*Use those which are compatible with client's needs and pause between each one.*)

I see clear and pure unconditional love, I love what I see and will it to happen...

I welcome a relationship which is fulfilling in all ways and the one created for me will find me...

I can feel the love my partner and I have for each other and it's growing stronger and stronger every day...

My partner and I are perfectly in tune with each other emotionally and physically...

My partner and I are fully compatible and perfectly aligned intellectually...

My partner and I are fully compatible and perfectly aligned spiritually...

My partner and I are perfectly in tune and sexually compatible...

I desire love and romance in my life; I draw love and romance into and my life and accept it now...

I am an enticing and irresistible to my partner...

I radiate pure, unconditional love towards my partner...

My partner and I are loyal to each other and our love continues to grow daily, weekly, monthly, yearly...

I draw love and romance into my life and I accept it now...

I am magnetic and irresistible to my partner...

I radiate pure, unconditional love towards my partner...

Love happens! I release the desperate need for love. I release the need for my partner to approve of me. I allow love to find me easily and effortlessly...

Love is all around me. I feel it everywhere. Joy fills my entire world...

My partner is the love of my life and we adore each other...

I now deserve love, romance, and joy...and all the blessings that life has to offer me...

I am safe in all my relationships. I am always treated well...

I am very grateful for all the love in my life. I find it everywhere...

My heart is open to love. I speak loving words to my partner and my partner speaks loving words to me...

I have a wonderful partner, and we are both happy and at

peace...

I am in a satisfying, intimate relationship with a person who truly loves me...

I laugh with my partner more and more each day...

I deserve love and sexual pleasure and provide the same in return...

I am now open and prepared to accept a happy, fulfilling relationship...

I am now drawing exactly the kind of relationship I want...

I am now divinely irresistible to my perfect mate...

I am open to receiving love and to extending it...

I interact with my partner positively and joyfully more and more each day...

Giving my partner unconditional love makes me feel energized...

I look for ways to contribute to my partner's growth and happiness. I support my partner in their goals unselfishly, knowing that it will make them happy...

I respect what my partner has to say. I listen to my partner with genuine interest...

I offer empathy when appropriate...

I desire love, so I give my partner love...

I desire respect, so I give my partner respect...

I desire cooperation, so I give my partner cooperation...

I desire compassion, so I give my partner compassion...

I desire control, so I give my partner control...

Now that you have put all your positives desires out there and know in your mind and heart these will take place exactly as you desire them to...I want you to imagine or visualize once again that you are with you partner...notice as you both are happy, relaxed, affectionate, showing all emotional feelings towards each other...notice and feel the unconditional love you have for each other...

Visualize and imagine as you both walk hand in hand, looking adoringly into each other's eyes...perhaps you are walking along the sea shore...notice that, each time the water laps over your feet, how your love for each other grows even stronger...Feel the closeness, feel the love between the both of you... (*pause*)

Let this image become stronger every day...as you open yourself more and more to the ideal relationship that you desire...that you deserve.

Exiting Script

by June Austin

Use this to prepare your client for surfacing and to embed post hypnotic suggestion for future sessions. Speak slowly and deliberately...

Today, you have learned some interesting things about how your mind, emotions and body are inter-connected and how they function best together for you. Today you have set in motion a process...that will create an environment to support and project you forward into a regarding and promising future. With this comes a renewed sense of positive self-appreciation and confidence in your ability to direct and navigate future events in your life successfully.

You have also re-discovered how your mind and body naturally release emotional and physical tension in a safe and comfortable way. From this moment forward, you will release the day's unfavourable tensions easily and automatically...each and every night as you sleep. When you prepare yourself for sleep each night, you will notice how quickly and effortlessly you glide into a dreamy slumber...that will completely rest your body, un-clutter your mind and support emotional balance. If you must awaken to attend to something important, you will do so with clear and alert attention. When you are finished with what must be done, you will simply drift back into a fully restful sleep.

From this day forward, you will awaken rejuvenated each morning, with an abundant supply of energy for the whole day. Your mind will be completely alert and focused and your emotions balanced. You will notice every day that you are becoming more confident, enthusiastic and experiencing

421

more joy in your life.

In a moment...but not yet...you will return to your daytime awareness...feeling refreshed and completely at ease. You have found this hypnotic experience to be pleasant and effective. You will likely continue to have more insights about yourself and your world between now and your next session with me.

When we meet again for your next appointment, you will achieve an even deeper and more profoundly effective level of hypnosis. Each and every time you are hypnotized, you will safely travel deeper...even deeper...than now...quickly and easily in this way:

Only with your permission, will I, or anyone else, be able to hypnotize you. I will secure the room and when you are ready, you will close your eyes...After a few cleansing breaths, I will slowly count down...from five...to one. When I reach the word "one", I will snap my fingers like this (*snap fingers or use any other preferred associative trigger like a knuckle rap on a hard surface, say "Sleep!", etc...*) You will then find that you have travelled ten times deeper into hypnosis that are...even at this moment.

We will then work again together to successfully redesign how you want to live daily life, or solve any mysteries or concerns until you have resolved them all and move confidently forward into your bright and rewarding future.

Alright, ready now...I will begin to count from one to five...at the count of five you will open your eyes, feeling rejuvenated, refreshed and completely relaxed. (*Emerge client*)

Contributor Submission Index

Directory of Hypnotic Women Authors

June Austin, CHt, Certified Dental Asst., Provincial Instructor, Reiki Mast, Singer/Song Writer in North Vancouver, NC, Canada. Currently in limited practice while in research and development. www.juneaustin.co, geminikrikit@telus.net.

Dawna Bailey (Hunter), MH, CCHt, Surrey, BC, Canada. Proud graduate of the Pacific Institute of Advanced Hypnotherapy, writer, publisher and mother with a strong, life-long desire to help others achieve healing and growth from the inside, out. InsideOut.CHt@gmail.com, 778-230-2230

Vivienne Barker, CCHt, working in Australia, specializing in smoking cessation. www.hypnosisworksmackay.com

Michelle Braun is a medical hypnotherapist, dementia therapy specialist and NLP practitioner located in San Diego County, CA. She has trance-formed her own life using hypnosis and NLP into one of ever increasing health and joy after having been poisoned by pesticides. www.ManifestIntent.com, 619-792-2068

Sue Bridgman, CCHt, Colorado. Director, Chocolate Blues Business Networking Festivals. Specializing in fun business networking and relationship building. www.Colorado@bizfestival.com, 970-405-4967

Helen Bremner, Registered Nurse Hypnotherapist in Worcester, Worchestershire, England. Integrative Hypnotherapy for Intensive Care, Colorectal and IBS. www.westmidlandshypnotherapy.webs.com ph:07779558829

Bev Bryant, CHt (retired), Everett, WA. Lover of dogs and President of the Animal Rescue Foundation.

Monika Burton, MH,CCHt, Vancouver, BC, Canada. Dolores Cannon Quantum Healing Hypnosis Professional. monikaburton@yahoo.com

Joanna Cameron, CHt, Stage Hypnotist (Trance Lady), McLean, VA
Time Line Therapy Trainer, Hypnosis Trainer, Member of American Board of Hypnotherapy, NGH.
Drjcameron@aol.com, www.joannacameron.com

Donna Carter, CCHt, Calistoga, CA
"Balanced change happens - Go ahead and read my name again".
www. calistogahypnosis.net, calistogahypnosis@live.com, 707-540-3080.

Michele Cempaka, CHt, Reiki Master, Transformational Coach in Denpasar, Bali, Indonesia. Michele provides transformative experiences for everyone she encounters. www.spiritweaverjourneys.com, mcempaka@gmail.com

Stephanie C. Conkle, CCHt, NLP, EFT, and Life Coach serving the Greater Atlanta, GA area. The author of "*Happy Person, Happy Life: A Recipe for Emotional Health and Well Being,*" and "*Land a Job using Hypnosis: Get the edge over your competitors*", her passion is helping others reach their fullest potential.
www.ClearLifeResults.com, 678-995-3549

Cynthia da Silva, BCH, Martha's Vineyard, MA In practice since 2003, Cynthia works with clients from around the world via phone or Skype and travels throughout the US offering workshops and private sessions.
www.dasilvahypnosis.com, 508.524.9022.

Shona Davenport Blackthorn, CHt, Victoria, Australia. Helping Others Help Themselves. www.southernhypnotherapy.com.au, 0411 281317

Camilla Edborg is a Hypnotherapist, Energy Healer and Mind-trainer, located in southern Sweden, Scandinavia. Her work is based on a holistic, body, mind, soul approach with the goal of achieving balance and finding happiness through self healing. www.ce-hypnosis.com, info@ce-hypnosis.com

Jagi Egnell, CCHt, Abbotsford, BC, Canada. Jagi works with people to empower them to create and fulfill their goals. www.hypnohealth@shaw.ca

Patricia Eslava Vessey, PCC, CCHt, ICF Credentialed Life & Executive Coach through the Intl. Coach Fed. and master practitioner of NLP with over 30 years exp. in social work. www.integritycoachingandtraining.com, Patricia@integritylifecoach.com, 206-459-2898

Carole Fawcett is a Professional Counsellor, Free-lance Writer and Clinical Hypnotherapist. She lives in the beautiful Okanagan Valley in British Columbia, Canada with her dog Chloe. www.amindfulconnection.com

Jackie Foskett, CHt and Hypno-Coach, Registered Dental Hygienist in the Seattle-Bellevue, WA area; Discover Your Inner Calm and Your Path to Your Best Life. www.HealingHypnotherapy.com, Jackie@JackieFoskett.com, 425-227-8210

Susan French, M.A., CCHt., in Tarzana, CA I've been practice for 12 years, specializing in anxiety disorders and addictions. www.hypno4success.com susanfrench2010@gmail.com, 888-333-3688.

Lorraine Gleeson, CCHt, Portsmouth, England, Hampshire School of Hypnotherapy, Author of *"How to be a Hypnotherapist"*. www.hsoh.co.uk

Zoilita Grant, Hypnotic Coach, Speaker, Teacher. Change Your Mind-Change Your Life! www.mindset-for-success.org, zoilita@zoilitagrant.net, 303-834-5040

Teya Graves, MH, CCHt, BC, Canada Specializing in eliminating fears and phobias. www.lakesidehypnotherapy.com, 604-703-9201

Iantha Greer, CCHt, Whitehorse, Yukon, Canada. Trained at the Pacific Institute for Advanced Hypnotherapy in Vancouver and owner of Indigo Hypnosis in Whitehorse.

Andrea Hedley, CCHt, Vancouver, BC, Canada. Get connected. Be inspired. Make profound change. www.shiftclinicalhypnotherapy.com, 604-264-0838

Angie J. Hernandez, CHt. Graduate of the Hypnosis Motivation Institute, Member Hypnotherapists Union Local 472 and the American Hypnosis Association. I specialize in helping you change your mind and life by phone, Skype or in person. www.IndianaHypnosis Center.com, 574-658-4686

Leta Heuer, CCHt, Certified Life Skills Coach and B.A.N.I. Childbirth Educator, Graduate of the Pacific Institute of Advanced Hypnosis. My practice, Salt of the Earth Coaching Services, is located in Swift Current, Saskatchewan, Canada. ledohypnotic@gmail.com

Sally Holmes Reed, CHt, Transformational Speaking Coach, Seattle, WA. Move out of past limitations and step into your bright new future. www.HypnosisSeattle.com, Sally@HypnosisSeattle.com, 206-719-6660

Sherry M. Hood, CCHt, Hypnotherapy Educator in New Westminster, BC, Canada. Owner of the Pacific Institute of Advanced Hypnotherapy: www.hypnotherapybc.com Sherry is also a private practitioner specializing in medical and clinical applications of hypnotherapy. ww.bchypnotherapy.com, hypnotic@shaw.ca, 778-397-7714

Jocelyn L.H. Jensen, CHt, Dip. Hyp., British Research and Training Institute. Ericksonian/Indirect Hypnosis specialist; in practice professionally since 1984. hypnosystemsuktherapy@inbox.com

Shannon King, CHt, Birthing as Nature Intended (B.A.N.I.) childbirth educator, and HOPE Coach, member of the IMDHA. Fall River Mills/Redding, CA area. Specializing in chronic pain and helping women heal from the trauma of abortion or miscarriage. www.heartofthematterhypnosis.com, 530-945-8319

Mary Lee LaBay, PhD, is the author of five books on hypnotherapy and past life regression, including *"Hypnotherapy: A Client-Centered Approach"*. She is the instructor of Bastyr University's non-credit Hypnotherapy Training Program, instructs Past Life Regression and spiritual applications of hypnosis elsewhere, and maintains a private practice in Bellevue, WA. www.maryleelabay.com, 425-562-7277

Heather Lauzon, CCHt, Vancouver Island, BC, Canada. You have always held the key to divine health; Emerald Healing Place will support you in your journey of reclaiming it! www.emeraldhealingplace.com, heather@emeraldhealingplace.com, 250-732-1405

Janice Lesley, Vancouver, BC, Canada www.janicelesley.com, 604-812-2159

Cindy Levy, LMHC, CCHt, MH (Stage Hypnosis), and Psychodrama Certification Candidate, Olympia, WA www.cindylevy.com, 360-888-6630

Vanessa Lindgren, CCHt, Northern Virginia, USA. Clinical Hypnotherapist specializing in medical hypnosis, in practice for 20 years. www.modernhypnosisworks.com, hypnosisdrvanessa@gmail.com, 540-454-0213

Toni Macri-Reiner, CHt, Faster EFT practitioner, Indianapolis, IN Change your mind...Change your life. www.Indianahypnosisforchange.com, 317-207-0537

Mariana A. Matthews, CCHt, Comedy Entertainer, Lecturer. Certified in a variety of subjects but most passionate in the belief that "Laughter is the BEST therapy." www.thatladyhypnotist.com, mariana@thatladyhypnotist.com, 425-248-7676

Kit Muehlman, CHt, Registered Yoga Teacher (RYT500), Mount Vernon, WA. My clients come for hypnotherapy modeled after wellness practices such as yoga, meditation and Ayurveda. www.kittravishypnosis.com

Rosi Nesaura, CHt and energy healer. Chicago and Palatine, IL Body, mind and soul heal all. 847-778-1305

Lani Nicholls, CCHt, Wellness Coach in Arlington, WA. Nearly 30 yrs experience of helping people connect with that place inside where wisdom and healing reside. www.laninichollshypnosis.com, laninicholls@gmail.com

Joy O'Dwyer, CCHt, Vancouver, BC,Canada. Mind Over Matter Clinical Hypnotherapy, www.vancouverhypnotherapy.yolasite.com

Vicky Ortiz, CCHt, with extended training in Past Life Regression, Registered Dental Hygienist, graduate of Pacific Institute of Advanced Hypnotherapy and member of IMDHA. Private practice located in Williams Lake, BC, Canada. vicortiz@netbistro.com, mindpathhypnosis@shaw.ca

Paula Reynolds, CCHt, Life Coach who helps people to work through issues so they can live the best life possible. www.essencehypnotherapy.ca essencehypnotherapy@hotmail.com.

Linda Roan, CHt, HOPE Coach, Biofeedback,Medical Hypnosis, Mindful Word/Art & Energy Practitioner in practice since 2001. Oakville, Ontario, CANADA www.insightconnections.ca, linda@insightconnections.ca, 416- 648-1290

Marion Robb, CCHt, Master NLP Practitioner in Edinburgh, Scotland, UK. A mentor for new hypnotherapists, Marion also is a referral specialist for Anxiety UK. www.conscious-choice.co.uk

Alina Robinson, MH, CCHt, Graduate of the Pacific Institute of Advanced Hypnotherapy, member of IMDHA, Certified Massage Provider. alinaeva55@gmail.com, 250-668-9908

Seth-Deborah Roth, RN,CRNA,CCHt,CI Fellow National Board of Certified Clinical Hypnotherapists, Instructor with the NGH, member of IMDHA. Castro Valley, CA Specializing in Medical Hypnosis: "Combining Medical Experience and Hypnosis is the Difference." www.HypnotherapyForHealth.com SethDeborah@HypnotherapyForHealth.com, 510-690-0699

Jeannie Lynn Rudyk, CCHt, RHN, CPT. Member IMDHA, Graduate of Pacific Institute of Advanced Hypnotherapy. Harmonic mind, holistic body.
www.Harmonicmind.ca, jeannierudyk@harmonicmind.ca

Doris Santic, CCHt, New Westminster, BC, Canada
doris.santic@gmail.com

Maria Sideris, CCHt, Vancouver and Fraser Valley, BC, Canada
Graduate of Pacific Institute of Advanced Hypnotherapy. 13 years experience working with children for social, emotional development.
604-343-1833

Ender Tanrikut, CCHt, Vancouver, BC, Canada
Specializing in pain management, anxiety, phobias and performance hypnosis, I also love to work with children and teenagers. www.successmindpower.com, 604-363-1203

Jodie Tessier, H.Ba, M.H., C.CHt. Counselor in Caledon, ON, Canada. PIAH graduate and member of the IMDHA. One Life, Unlimited New Beginnings.
www.pfhypno.com, pfhypno@gmail.com

Sheila Wardman, CHt, Eagle Bay, BC, Canada
Creating and Inspiring Powerful Lives by Design!
www.inperfecthealth.ca, sheila@inperfecthealth.ca, 250-517-9690

Monique Wilson, CCHt, Maple Ridge, BC, Canada
Achieving Peace of Mind. www.achievingpeaceofmind.com, 604-462-8220

Kelley T. Woods, Hypnotist and HOPE Coach in Mount Vernon, WA
www.woodshypnosis.com, www.mindfulhypnosiscoach.com

Birgit Wujcik, CHt, Spruce Grove, Alberta, Canada. Success is achieving a goal you set yourself that starts with a simple thought; where you supply the thought and I help you clear the way to success. www.hypnosisforsuccess.ca

Katherine Zimmerman, CCHt, Director of the California Hypnotherapy Academy. Offering continuing education for hypnotherapists since 1994.
www.trancetime.com, info@trancetime.com

Made in the USA
San Bernardino, CA
22 March 2014